MIND YOUR MOVEMENT

Laura V. Dow

ISBN: 979-8-9903513-1-8 (paperback)

ISBN: 979-8-9903513-2-5 (Ebook)

Cover design, spine and back cover by David Deakin, www.daviddeakin.com

Book production by Scriptor Publishing Group, www.scriptorpublishinggroup.com

Editing by Seth Arenstein

Author photograph Matt Mendelsohn, www.mattmendelsohn.com

Interior photographs Tori Fuller and Rachael Foster

Praise for *Mind Your Movement*

"Laura Dow has written an ideal handbook to help adults move from feeling stiff and out of shape to achieving fitness, well-being, strength, and optimal health. Her model is comprehensive and well thought out and she walks you through the stages to getting strong and fortifying your body, mind, and spirit, one step at a time. Unlike many exercise programs, Laura has created a targeted roadmap to wellness that features building blocks that will not overwhelm you, but instead are simple steps that propel you to strength, wellbeing, and a profound feeling of truly being fit."

Gail McMeekin, LICSW,
career and creativity coach and author of multiple books including "The 12 Secrets of Highly Successful Women."

"This book spoke right to the heart of the matter – YES, our aging bodies can still move! All you need to do is read this book to gain the motivation, intention and mindset to get going beginning today. The frankness and practicality of this book is a testament to Laura's skill, heart and mind in working with her older clients. I am one. And have been her devoted client for many of my senior years. This book is a necessary roadmap for any senior adult who wants to get moving again and get FIT! No matter what your age is."

Susan Cherney

"Laura offers foundational wisdom to anyone who is ready (or almost ready) to get more engaged with the body and enjoy the whole-life benefits of moving more mindfully and moving more consistently."

Nicole M. Seitz,
Psychotherapist

"I thought I knew quite a bit about the human body, specifically my own, since I have been physically active most of my life and have a medical background. However, after reading this enlightening book, I realized I had forgotten the basics that can lead to a healthy lifestyle and help with aging. Laura provides simple exercises, along with illustrations of correct body mechanics that are absolutely needed for an improved body, as well as an improved mental attitude. Particularly, the sections on correct posture, ability to balance to help reduce the risk of a fall, and different breathing techniques to deal with life were so illuminating to me! I had forgotten those basics that are necessary to have a healthy body and mind. I highly recommend this book to those wanting to learn how to begin to improve their lifestyles and to "athletes" who need to refresh their memories on the basics of healthy living."

Mary Ann D, R.N.,
Assistant Director for Health (retired)

★★★★★ (5/5)

"Mind Your Movement" is an absolute gem for anyone looking to improve senior mobility. As a woman in my early 30s, I found it incredibly valuable not only for preparing for my own future but also for my role as a caregiver. The exercises are easy to follow, with clear instructions and helpful illustrations. I particularly loved the balance exercises—they're practical and safe, making a real difference in preventing falls.

The holistic approach, covering not just physical fitness but also mental well-being and nutrition, makes this book a standout. It's inspiring to read the personal stories and see how others have benefited.

I highly recommend "Mind Your Movement" to anyone in the senior community, those caring for older adults, or anyone looking to prepare for a healthy future. It's practical, encouraging, and full of valuable tips!

Valeria L.,
Small Business Coach

Well-written, inviting and pleasurable, "Mind Your Movement" immediately engaged my attention and is a wonderful reframe of what is often a preachy, threatening topic-EXERCISE!

By reading this book, I realized my body is not getting as much attention as my mind and spirit during my daily life. I appreciate the author's acknowledgement of accepting wherever the reader is at with their fitness level as well as the client vignettes and the author's own story which were easy to identify with and relatable.

Martha S.,
Founder & Owner, Hearts & Hands Reiki

MIND YOUR MOVEMENT

Six Essential Physical and Mental Tools To Stay Active As You Age

Laura V. Dow

BA, MM, CPT & RYT-500

Master Personal Trainer

Registered Yoga Teacher

Certified Nutrition & Wellness Coach

Pilates Integrated Movement Specialist

Certified Senior Fitness, Orthopedic and Corrective Exercise Specialist

Subject Matter Expert for Job Task Analysis Project, American College of Sports Medicine

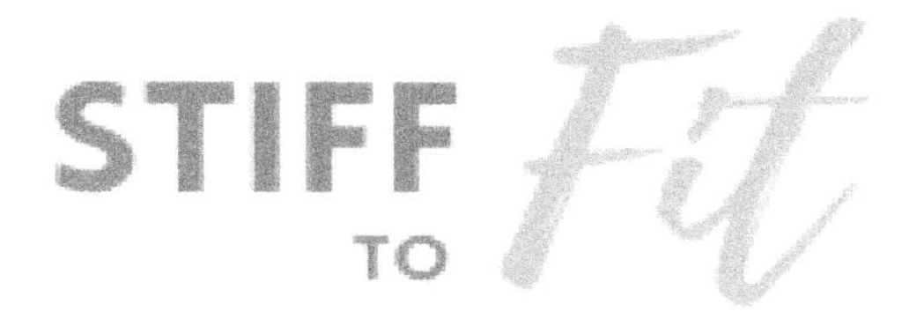

www.StifftoFit.com

"Whether you think you can or you think you can't, you're right"

Henry Ford (1863-1947)
American industrialist and Founder,
Ford Motor Company

"Now I Become Myself"

May Sarton (1912-1995)
Belgian American author and poet

Let July be July.
Let August be August.

And let yourself

just be

even in

the uncertainty.

You don't have to fix

everything.

You don't have to solve

everything.

And you can still

find peace

and grow

in the wild

of changing things.

Morgan Harper Nichols (born 1990)
American Christian musician, songwriter,
mixed-media artist, and writer

Table of Contents

Introduction

What's your daily movement like?

Do you think about what your body needs or as I like to call it, "your self-care"?

Do your mind and body work together as a team or are they on opposing sides?

Are you satisfied with how you're living in your body?

If not, "*Mind Your Movement, 6 Essential Physical and Mental Tools to Stay Active As You Age*" may be a useful guide for you with information, explanation and tips for better movement and self-care.

Staying active and living independently are life goals for most of us, particularly as we age.

Understanding basic movement principles and **how** to stay active is time well spent.

In some cases, doing so may mean the difference between living the way you want or needing physical assistance.

Besides information, tips and ideas to increase your physical activity, this book also includes client stories.

Reading someone else's story may help us recognize that we all have challenges and obstacles to overcome to get enough movement and physical activity.

You can use some of the strategies mentioned in these stories or maybe you will come up with your own solution. One key point to understand is it's possible to improve.

I am an example of the ideas contained in this book.

Here is my story:

Laura's Story

My journey to better movement and health includes many starts and stops.

Perhaps you can relate.

Like other women of my generation, growing up, I did not have access to organized sports and did not pursue sports in college.

In the mid-1980's I belonged to a Jane Fonda-inspired, women-only gym where I used 3lb pink weights for most of the exercises. I also played weekend tennis, biked and hiked.

As often happens, due to marriage, work and change of careers, my physical activities took a back seat to these other areas. I gained weight in the early 90's, then somewhat serendipitously got involved in martial arts, started jogging and joined a gym to do weight training.

With these physical activities, I got fit(er) and lost 50 lbs in the late 90's. Unfortunately, I also got injured due to overtraining and gained 65 lbs in the early 2000's.

During these years, feeling confident meant a specific number on the scale or a particular dress size.

Through martial arts, I began to question my previous self-identity as a "non-athlete." But I still didn't appreciate or understand what my body could do for me. I only knew the number on the scale and my dress size didn't conform to society's ideals and therefore my body and by extension, I, was bad.

Getting injured running, dealing with multiple lower leg issues taking months to heal, regaining more weight than I had lost and not being able to exercise during my injuries, were major blows to my health and self-esteem.

At this point, I was in my early forties and working as a professional musician. I was significantly overweight, unhealthy, unhappy and sedentary.

After multiple attempts at trying to lose weight myself, I decided to hire several professionals, including health-care providers and a personal trainer.

By my mid-forties, I was in a much healthier and happier state, exercising regularly and had lost 75 lbs. I was also reassessing my life.

An unintended consequence of my personal fitness journey resulted in moving to California and becoming a personal trainer.

In 2005, fitness in California seemed to me to be solely represented by tanned, toned, lithe, young blonde humans. That's a stereotype, of course. But as a middle-aged woman on her personal fitness path, I felt out of place.

While I continued my routine at a health club in Northern California, I also began working as an assistant at a female-only gym. The owners of the gym asked me to get certified as a trainer to help their members, which began my fitness career.

After that health club closed, I continued as a personal trainer and group fitness instructor in commercial big box gyms in Marin, San Francisco and later Washington, DC.

I was almost always the only "older woman trainer," often by several decades. Many of my younger, male colleagues had participated in organized sports, as had some of the females. They wore the label "athlete" easily.

Even though my martial arts experience showed me I had athletic abilities and I successfully competed at the state level in martial arts tournaments, I did not relate to the idea of being an athlete.

I felt like a unicorn and an outlier.

Being a unicorn meant I stuck out, which I came to realize was not necessarily bad. Older women who didn't want to work with younger trainers quickly found me and my business grew.

These women didn't want to hire someone who didn't or couldn't appropriately adapt exercising for an aging woman's body. As an older female myself, I already shared common ground with them.

Being an outlier also meant that I began to develop different ideas about working with women.

Training females meant modifying exercises to their bodies, NOT forcing their bodies to conform to fitness ideals.

Clients uniformly wanted to feel better and move better; to stay active and independent. Many were recovering from an injury or were post-surgery/post-rehab for joint replacements.

Having suffered my own set of injuries, I understood their goals.

Throughout this time, my perspective on weight, body image and dress sizes changed dramatically. I became appreciative of how strong I was and what my body could do, rather than berating it for not conforming to a particular shape or weighing a certain number.

My training also evolved over the years. Instead of emphasizing numbers or dress size, I focused on health, well-being and how clients feel in their bodies. I also stressed agency and self-efficacy, the idea that clients were capable of instituting successful change in their lives, in movement and other areas.

I was and am terrifically proud of my clients for their commitment to themselves and to their bodies. We celebrate every push-up, squat and plank. Sometimes just showing up is an act of courage.

Helping people understand their bodies and teaching them how to move better and feel better is my passion. We all can improve how we live in our bodies, regardless of our knowledge and previous exercise experience.

This book is a love letter to the people I've had the privilege and honor to work with, whether for an hour or many years. Every client and yoga class member has contributed to my growth as a fitness professional.

I am now in my mid-60's and have been a fitness professional for more than 20 years yet I am still on my fitness journey. As I age, I modify my exercise routine according to what my body needs while understanding that movement and strength are vital to live life the way I want to.

I also reassess and recommit to my self-care regularly. Sometimes these are very conscious decisions and other times my body alerts me to move.

"Oh, I've been sitting for too long; my back is stiff and I'm hunching my shoulders. Time to walk and to stretch."

While I have the same goals as clients to stay active and live independently, I also recognize that nobody, me included, is guaranteed those outcomes.

Bad things happen, no matter how much we may try to get it "right."

I do my best to appreciate what my body can do today, this week and this month, knowing that my physical abilities can and will change as I age.

Regular movement, lifting weights, rest and recovery, proper sleep, eating healthy food and drinking enough water give me a better chance of living my life the way I want to and reducing the risk of injury or falling.

I'm sharing my story so it's clear that I've experienced issues with exercise, injuries and overtraining.

I often tell clients I've made every mistake a person can make about exercising.

That's an exaggeration but I've made many, many mistakes. I want you to know I'm human and share my story in the hopes you avoid my errors.

This book, "*Mind Your Movement*" is an extension of my own experience with better movement and getting fit(er) as well as my professional work training clients over a 20-year career.

I hope you can utilize the information presented to move better and feel better.

HOW THIS BOOK IS ORGANIZED

In the book, Chapters 1-4 offer foundational physical concepts with a brief explanation about how your body operates. In chapters 5-7, I include tips on getting your mind and body to work together as equal partners.

The purpose of this book is to:

- Provide educational and immediately applicable information
- Increase confidence about your self-care
- Use your mind in service to your body

Each chapter focuses on a specific element, offering a basic explanation of the idea, physical tools and mental tips. Throughout the book are also client stories and a few "Deeper Dive" sections, which dig into the material more, providing additional information.

Caution sections are also provided, alerting readers to issues that could lead to mistakes. I close each chapter with a Keep It Simple prompt, short recaps of the previous content.

About the client stories: though the stories are based on actual clients, I've created composites in most cases and disguised names in all the stories to protect their privacy.

INFORMATION

We are continually bombarded with a vast amount of health and fitness information, often contradictory, on how to move better, feel better, live better.

It's a lot of work to sift through the information and to determine what's useful.

Most people do not have the time, energy or desire to educate themselves on basic human movement and how to improve their own movement.

This book focuses on key concepts so you can understand your body better and more importantly, get you moving.

While "*Mind Your Movement*" is written with each chapter building on the previous one, the chapters also present stand-alone ideas.

For instance, if you're most interested in balance, you can focus just on that chapter. Or you may prefer to use the physical tools rather than the mental tips.

You can start at the beginning, open the book in the middle or read the last chapter first. You can skim or skip the Deeper Dive sections or use the resources to pursue a concept even more.

Perhaps a second reading gets you interested in a topic you had previously skimmed or an idea in the Deeper Dive section catches your eye.

Use the book however it works best for you.

I chose to limit the scope of "*Mind Your Movement*" to basic physical activities of the human body which, done regularly, will help you stay active and move better.

Therefore, several important topics-nutrition, hydration, sleep to name a few are not explored.

Understanding the movement ideas is critical but acting on the information and tips presented, as best suits you, is even more vital.

Receiving useful information without subsequent action is almost the same as not receiving any information at all.

You may have a thousand reasons why you don't act.

However, change is NOT possible without some kind of step forward, metaphorically and literally.

Mind Your Movement is not a book of directions, "you must do this; you must do that."

Instead, I am offering you information about human movement and giving you a guide on how to change.

You are responsible for your body and you get to decide which step to take.

If you want change, i.e., more movement and physical activity, action is mandatory.

However, large commitments of time, money and energy are not necessary to get started (or to keep moving).

Be assured that small steps, taken consistently over time, can yield big results.

Here's an easy visual for this idea:

Knowledge + Consistent Action/Over Time = Results

This equation is powerful, simple AND it works.

We'll get to how to implement the idea in Chapter 5 "Mind".

Understand that you do NOT have to become an elite athlete or Olympian to move better and get fit(er).

We sometimes hear stories of older adults achieving incredible physical results and tend to view such achievements as superhuman. Many of us don't relate and think "Well, not me."

But wait.

I'm **not** saying you must go to the gym every day, stand on your head or ski a black diamond run to get fit(er).

I **AM** stating that whatever your physical situation, you ***can*** improve.

Many of us have aches, pains or even serious medical ailments which may prevent us from moving well.

Perhaps we have non-physical constraints such as caring for family members or other types of challenges.

Each of us has life situations which might limit our ability to move.

Therefore, our improvement will look different than someone else's.

You are unique.

Your body and physical circumstances are unique.

I don't know what's possible for you, but I do know there's some element or several elements of movement which you can improve.

Research continues to show that with regular physical activity, most older adults can improve their health, general fitness and well-being.

Health indicators such as cardiac and respiratory status, muscle strength and endurance, body composition (fat vs. lean muscle mass) and metabolism are all positively affected by consistent exercise, leading to better health and movement.

You may not run a sub-3-hour marathon at age 65, be a champion body builder at 75 or set a world record for rowing at 95. As stated previously, you may have an illness or injury that affects how your body moves.

Still, change is possible.

Ask yourself again: Are you satisfied with how you're living in your body?

If yes, I applaud you and say, "Keep going!"

If not, I want to give you hope and encouragement that you *can* change how you live in your body.

And why is moving so important? I know some of you would rather sit on the couch, watch TV and get your steps as you walk to the fridge and back for a snack.

But every function in your body involves movement. Your lungs move as you breathe, your heart pulses, digestion is continuous movement, even your brain emits waves. Your sleep also occurs as waves and your blood moves through your body in waves.

Physical movement is a continuation of the way the body already operates. Not only does physical activity supports body functions, but daily movement also improves mood and mental concentration.

According to a Mintel Study, most people who exercise (78%) do so primarily for their mental/emotional well-being. And 89% of peer-reviewed research found a positive, statistically significant relationship between exercise/physical activity and mental health.

https://www.mintel.com/press-centre/in-person-gyms-to-make-a-comeback-as-only-15-of-us-exercisers-feel-digital-platforms-have-eliminated-the-need-for-gyms/

Movement literally is life.

After reading *Mind Your Movement*, you should have a stronger physical and mental foundation to live better in your body as well as ideas on how to get your body and mind working more in partnership.

Positive change is possible at whatever age you may be.

Before You Begin

I am not an expert on your body.

In writing for a general audience, I do not address specific medical conditions, injuries or personal histories.

I am not a therapist or mental health professional.

The tools and tips in this book, while gentle and straight-forward, are simply ideas for you to consider.

Before implementing any of these suggestions, evaluate whether an idea in this book is right for you and always consult with medical professionals.

Let's begin.

1 BREATH

"Breathe in deeply to bring your mind home to your body."

Thich Nhat Hanh (1926-2022)
Vietnamese Buddhist monk, author and peace activist

"Listen...are you breathing just a little, and calling it a life?"

Mary Oliver (1935-2019)
American Poet

BREATH

Why begin a book about movement with a discussion of breathing?

Did you think I would already be shouting at you to get off the couch and start moving?

Not so fast.

If you think breathing just happens, that you've lived this long without instructions on breathing so no further directions are necessary and you'll just skip ahead to the next chapter, consider this statement:

Breathing is movement.

Your lungs expand as you inhale, your lungs contract as you exhale.

Or put another way, breathing is a cycle of inhaling and exhaling.

And breathing is essential to being alive and important to moving well.

As stated above, breathing is a constant cycle of ebb and flow, expansion/contraction, pulse and stillness. Ocean waves are a good analogy. Picture the movement of tides with the water rushing forward and then receding. I think all of us would agree that waves are water in action.

Similarly, your breath is a continuous ebb and flow of air, at least during your lifespan.

This ebb and flow of air creates physical movement in the body.

You breathe in, your body expands to accommodate the inflow of air. Breathe out and your body contracts to release the by-products of your inhale as you prepare for the next breath.

Need a visual?

Take a moment and watch Jessica Wolf's incredible animated video that demonstrates how the body operates during the breath cycle.

https://www.youtube.com/watch?v=SAk77hTiwtY

Breathing well does more than create movement in the body. Breathing positively affects:

- Mood
- Digestion
- Vitality (perception of physical energy)
- Concentration & attention among other bodily functions.

Breathing better is always possible (unless you have a medical condition affecting your cardio-respiratory system). For instance, breathing more slowly and deeply can generate positive results in our bodies such as making exercise easier, feeling calmer after a difficult conversation, or improving concentration for an urgent task.

And breathing is free!

You don't need a gym, expensive sneakers, the latest fitness gadget, pricey gym clothes or a dedicated work out area.

Maybe you've lived this long without paying much attention to your breathing (except for huffing and puffing up the stairs?).

But, by understanding how to breathe better, you have the possibility of feeling and moving better.

If you haven't paid much attention to your breath, no worries. You can start now by reviewing Wolf's video and noticing how the body moves throughout the breath cycle.

Whether you chose to spend time on breathing or not, note that the worst scenario is holding your breath which sounds crazy but is more common than you think.

Jane's story, a little later in this chapter, demonstrates how not breathing while "trying hard" can get in the way of moving well.

In the meantime, here are 2 short exercises to help you tune in to your breathing.

Exercise #1

To repeat: breathing is a cycle of exhale, inhale, exhale, inhale. These waves of breath create physical change in the body that we can feel if we pay attention.

Whether you're seated, standing or reclining, inhale and notice any movement in your body. You may feel movement in your torso, perhaps a sense of expansion as you inhale.

If you watched Wolf's video, you'll remember that during an inhalation, the rib cage flares outward as the body creates room for the inflow of air.

Now exhale and notice any movement in your body. You may feel your torso contracting. While exhaling, the body responds by using muscles to expel the by-products from the inhale (primarily CO2). Your rib-cage moves in and down, returning to its original position before the next inhale.

Continue with 3-5 breath cycles. See if you can feel your body moving during both phases of your breath-inhale and exhale.

Exercise #2

Having trouble feeling any physical sensations?

An easy way to become more aware of your breath is to lie on the floor on your back if you can get down to the floor and back up again safely. Your knees can be bent or straight, either works although most folks prefer their knees to be bent to support their back.

Put both your hands on your belly. Inhale and see if you can feel your hands move up toward the ceiling or out toward the sides. Find an easy flow of in breath and out breath and keep this flow going for a minute or two.

Stop and assess.

How do you feel?

Most people report a greater sense of relaxation physically and a mental calmness or slowing of their minds.

If you don't feel your hands moving, try putting a medium size book on your belly. Can you get the book to lift toward the ceiling on your inhale? And does the book lower back down on your exhale?

If yes, that's it.

Here's an example:

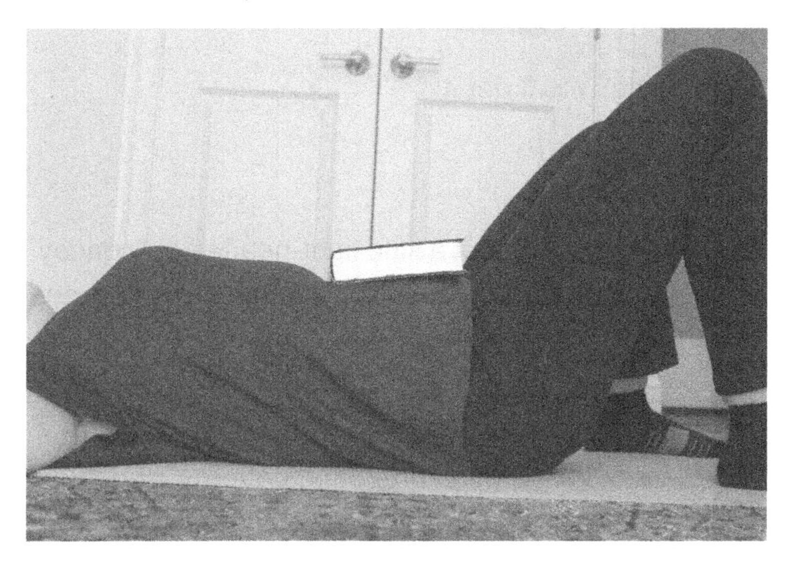

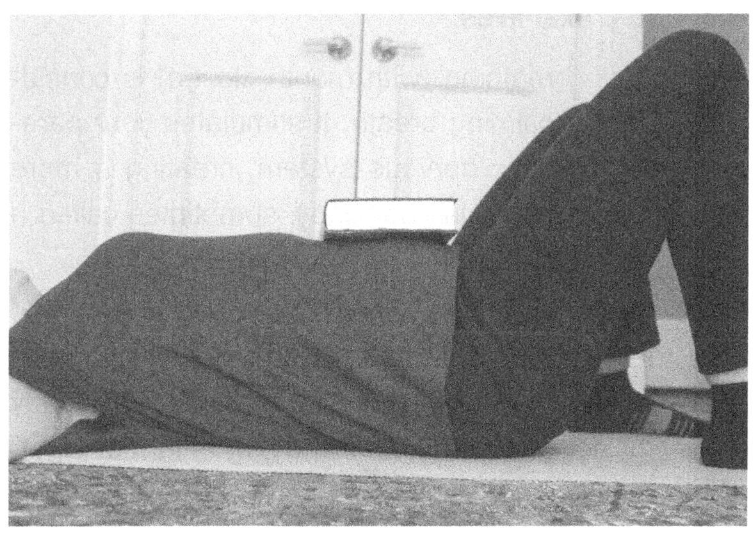

Becoming more aware of your breathing takes practice.

Keep trying. You'll get it.

CAUTION

Sometimes people feel a little light-headed or "spacey" when they consciously breathe like this. Be smart and safe. Take your time getting up.

Deeper Dive

There are many types of breathing patterns, and those individual patterns affect the body differently.

Here are 3 examples:

1. Nose breathing (with mouth closed) is considered a calming breath. It stimulates your parasympathetic nervous system, creating a more relaxed state in your body, sometimes called a "rest and digest" reaction in yoga.
2. Mouth breathing, when you inhale and exhale through your mouth, activates your sympathetic nervous system, creating a more excited, ready for action state in your body, the "fight or flight" reaction.

3. Sighing (a vocalized exhale with an open mouth) can often help us more fully expel air and may release shoulder and neck tension.

Knowing what type of breathing is calming and what type is excitatory can be very useful in exercising as well as in life.

If you're running, breathing with your mouth results in more air filling your lungs more quickly, much needed when your body is working hard.

If you're taking a yoga class, breathing through your nose with mouth closed may be the most effective way to stay present to your body.

In life, if you're nervous about starting a meeting, slow nose breathing might help calm you. If you're feeling sleepy right before a test, mouth breathing might energize you and allow you to focus better.

As in the running example, most exercise typically utilizes mouth breathing. Mouth breathing permits us to take in a bigger quantity of air quicker than nose breathing.

For breathing during exercise, specific breath patterns are recommended during most exercises, meaning you inhale at certain points and exhale at others. Breathing correctly will produce a more optimal result, often helping you perform the exercise better.

Usually, you exhale on the harder part of the exercise and inhale during the less difficult part. It can be tricky figuring out what part is hard and what part is easy(er).

Maybe all parts of the exercise seem hard to you. I understand.

A fitness professional can help you with when, how and where to breathe during specific exercises.

Because we often default to breathing through our mouths, nose breathing can feel unfamiliar. If you have asthma or severe allergies, you may feel that nose breathing is not an option.

Evaluate your situation and be thoughtful as to whether you want to try a different breathing pattern.

Mental Tip/Visualization

Here's a visualization that might help you with nose breathing:

Imagine something cooking that's delicious to you, maybe the smell of baking bread, a turkey roasting or chocolate chip cookies baking.

Maybe the smell of freshly brewed coffee, freshly cut grass or a beautiful cologne is more enticing for you. Pick whatever seems most luscious to you, imagine that smell and sniff it up through your nose keeping your mouth closed. Fully inhale that wonderful aroma.

Nose breathing is an excellent tool to calm your central nervous system. It allows your mind to stop being on high alert, scanning for saber-toothed tigers or horrible pandemics lurking about.

But what about the person (maybe you?) who has no awareness of their breathing or worse, holds their breath during exercise?

Here's a short client vignette about Jane, not breathing and "trying too hard."

Client Story

Concentration Face

Jane scrunched up her face in a tight scowl, pursed her lips, clenched her jaw and held her breath as she started the new exercise I had just given her. I asked if she was in pain. "No," she replied. Yet her face was telling me a different story. Jane said it was just "my concentration face." To me, Jane's concentration face looked tense and rigid.

More importantly, Jane didn't realize she was holding her breath.

Your back IS involved in breathing so imagining your breath as 3-dimensional (front of body, sides of body, back of body) can be importantly, she didn't realize she was holding her breath.

Besides keeping Jane alive, an even flow of breathing can help her better manage her work outs. Exhaling and inhaling at specific points during exercise can make movements feel easier.

Here's an example: picking up a box off the floor. The harder part is lifting the box, the easier part is lowering the body down to eventually lift the box. To correctly lift the box, inhale and lower the body, exhale and lift the box off the floor.

If Jane exhales as she lifts, that breathing pattern helps her pick up the weight more safely and with greater ease.very useful in learning to breathe better.

Besides keeping Jane alive, an even flow of breathing helps manage exercising. Exhaling and inhaling at specific points also makes movements feel easier.

Here's an example: picking up a box off the floor. The easier part is lowering the body down to the floor. The harder part is lifting the box off the floor as well as straightening the body to its original standing position.

To correctly lift the box, inhale and lower the body, exhale and lift the box off the floor.

Similarly, if Jane exhales as she lifts a weight during an exercise, that breathing pattern will help her pick up the weight more safely and with greater ease.

On the other hand, Jane's "concentration face" is unhelpful during exercise. Tightening her face wastes energy and pulls on other muscles in Jane's neck and upper back, potentially causing a negative chain reaction of tight muscles throughout the body.

The body perceives exercise as stress, which we sense as effort and tension. This type of stress is an appropriate reaction to increased workload like picking up a heavy bag of groceries off the floor.

Breathing properly helps you (and your body) manage the stress of exercise more effectively. Breathing incorrectly or worse, holding your breath, adds more stress during exercise which is not helpful and may be potentially harmful.

For Jane, she needs to become aware of the proper amount of effort and tension in the correct muscles.

When Jane tightened her facial muscles, her sensation of a tight face tricked her into thinking she was doing the exercise correctly.

If Jane's doing a leg exercise and all she feels is her face, something is very wrong.

And if Jane continues to hold her breath, she is not helping her body manage the stress of exercising. She may even inflict harm on herself unintentionally.

After Jane and I discussed her concentration face, she said tightening her face and holding her breath were long-term habits, an unconscious reaction that occurred when she exerted herself during exercise and other life activities.

What's the answer?

In Jane's case, getting her to think about breathing was the first step. Once I saw that she stopped holding her breath and began breathing more evenly, I asked Jane to create more space between her top and bottom teeth. This would help prevent her jaw from clenching. After becoming more aware of her jaw, I asked Jane to think "happy thoughts" during exercise.

That suggestion was not well received.

Instead, we settled on Jane working toward having a more neutral face.

Over time, Jane's breathing became automatic during exercise. Moreover, she was able to release most of the tension from her face and learned where in her body she should feel the effort of exercise.

Do you have a concentration face?

If you don't know, ask a friend, family member or co-worker.

They'll tell you.

If you do scrunch up your face in a scowl, furrow your brow and clench your jaw, whether you're exercising or not, you may want to consider some changes.

Remember, first become aware of how you're breathing. If you observe yourself holding your breath during any activity (not just exercise), immediately exhale and then inhale. Try to find an even flow of breath.

Breaking the habit of holding your breath may take time, so be kind and patient with yourself. It takes many repetitions to change a habit.

One repetitive action might be to send yourself reminders to breathe. You can use alerts on your phone or your laptop. Post-it Notes might be old school but they work too.

If you notice that you're breathing opposite to a trainer's cues or an instructor's cues in a group exercise class, no worries, that's fairly common. Better to breathe opposite an instructor's cues than to not breathe at all.

Try the breathing patterns suggested above and see what works for you.

The bottom line: You must breathe during exercise. The mental tips below may help.

Mental Tip #1 Remember the animated video? As you try the physical breathing tips, see if you can visualize Wolf's video, particularly how the rib cage moves during breath.

Here's the link again:

https://www.youtube.com/watch?v=SAk77hTiwtY

Seeing her video in your mind may help you better experience the physical movements during breathing.

Mental Tip #2 Become aware of your breathing. You can start anywhere. For instance, notice the next breath you take while reading this book. Observe your breathing while you go about your day. Waiting at a red light is a perfect time to focus on your breath.

Breathing can be disrupted when you're upset/annoyed/frustrated or upon hearing bad news.

We may have experienced jagged breathing, gasping or sometimes no breathing ourselves in such situations.

Becoming more observant of your breath is a positive step towards more optimal breathing. Once you've observed your breathing over time, you will be better able to intentionally choose your breathing pattern.

The first step is always observation and awareness.

Deeper Dive

If you tried the physical breathing tools listed previously, you may have sensed movement in your abdominal area when you breathe. If so, that's great.

But understand you are not breathing with your belly.

Instead, breathing happens in the lungs-they are the major organs of respiration.

The term **belly breathing,** which we hear so often, is factually incorrect.

There are no lungs in your belly. All breathing happens within the respiratory system, which the belly is NOT part of although you may feel your belly moving.

Likewise, you may have heard the term **diaphragmatic breathing**.

The diaphragm is the primary muscle in respiration, located under the lungs, slightly above the middle part of your torso. (remember the lungs are organs, not muscles).

Your diaphragm is an involuntary muscle, which means you cannot feel it or control it.

Because it's involuntary, you are always breathing with your diaphragm. In normal human life, there's no "non-diaphragmatic" breathing.

Like belly breathing, banish "diaphragmatic breathing" from your brain. It's redundant and misleading. All types of breathing involve movement of the diaphragm.

Since the diaphragm moves during the breath cycle, it affects other parts of your body that you CAN feel, like your abdomen. Therefore, you may be able to sense belly, back or chest movements during an inhale and exhale.

Sensing movement in the belly is usually the first step towards understanding how the body must expand to receive air during inhalation and how it contracts to expel air during exhalation.

You may also feel movement on the sides of the rib-cage as well as your back.

Think of your breath as a 3-dimensional process involving movement in the front and back and on the sides of your torso.

Wolf's video shows how the breath cycle creates a cascade of motion within the body.

As mentioned above, there are many types of breathing patterns (nose breathing, mouth breathing, alternate nostril breathing, fast breathing, shallow breathing). The diaphragm is active in every one of these.

Respiratory illness such as COPD and emphysema may cause altered breathing patterns. Some traumatic injuries can cause diaphragm paralysis. These situations may necessitate mechanical assistance to breathe, however, in most humans, the diaphragm requires no help to function properly.

We rarely focus on our breathing unless there's a problem, so most people spend very little, if any, time thinking about breath.

If you've read this far, congrats! I hope you have a new understanding and appreciation for the way breathing can positively affect our bodies. Breathing well has many physical and mental benefits.

I've presented several different physical exercises and mental tips to help you become better aware of your breath.

There are more.

If this is a topic of interest to you, consider attending a yoga class whether in person or online. Most yoga classes emphasize breathing and depending on the class, you'll learn different patterns and how each affects the body.

KEEP IT SIMPLE

Just breathe.

Sense the flow of air moving in your body.

Slow and steady wins the race.

2 POSTURE

"Do not lose your knowledge that our proper estate is an upright posture, an intransigent mind and a step that travels unlimited roads."

Ayn Rand (1905-1982)
Russian American author and philosopher

When I mention posture to clients, they tend to immediately rearrange themselves in a ramrod or military-like position, throw their chest forward and shoulders back, freeze like a statue and often display a terrified look on their faces.

Were you nagged as a child to "stand up straight, no slouching"?

I define posture a little differently.

Posture is optimal alignment of our body parts depending on what we're doing at that moment, whether we're upright or seated, stationary or moving.

It's a **dynamic process**, not a frozen position. If you're standing still, your body alignment will be different than if you're moving, for example.

When we're walking or running, alignment of the body changes as your body weight shifts during movement.

If you're seated, your posture could be different than when you're standing, depending on what you're doing as you're sitting.

Gravity is a factor, as it affects the body in every position.

But why should you care about good posture?

Like breathing, you may think that since you've made it to this point in your life with whatever posture you have, why bother to examine this now?

That perspective puts you in the majority.

A 2019 national survey by Orlando Health found that more than 50% of participants who completed the survey reported they were not concerned about poor posture or about the effects of poor posture on their health.

Should we move on to the next topic?

Absolutely not.

Instead, let's learn what poor posture does over time to the human body.

Nathaniel Melendez, an exercise physiologist at Orlando Health's National Training Center says:

"People don't realize the strain they're putting on their body when it is not aligned correctly, or just how far corrective exercises and daily adjustments can go toward improving pain and postural issues. Stretching your head forward of your body while texting on a cell phone, scrolling through social media or working at a computer puts tremendous pressure on your body. Even moving your head forward of your body 1 inch puts an extra 10lbs of pressure on your shoulders and upper back."

Melendez continues, "If, for example, your head is four inches in front of your body when you're looking down at your phone, that's like having a child sitting on your shoulders that whole time."

Oof!

Do you really want a child sitting on your shoulders?

The ubiquitous cell phone is the leading cause of forward head position although reading a book or working on a laptop can also result in a mal-aligned head posture.

Over time, holding one's head in this position leads to all kinds of issues such as neck pain, shoulder and low back pain to name a few.

Other common postures contributing to pain and long-term issues include:

- Hunching
- Slouching
- Caving the chest down and forward

Bad posture can result from sitting at a computer screen all day, attending endless Zoom meetings back-to-back or the daily scroll through social media or news on our cell phones.

Look at this excellent animated video on posture created by physical therapist Dr. Murat Dalkilinç. It's a wonderful demonstration of the points made by Nathaniel Melendez mentioned above and well worth putting this book down to watch.

https://www.youtube.com/watch?v=OyK0oE5rwFY

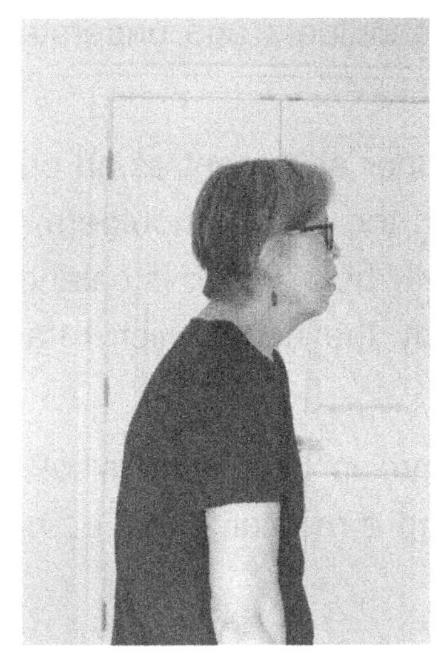
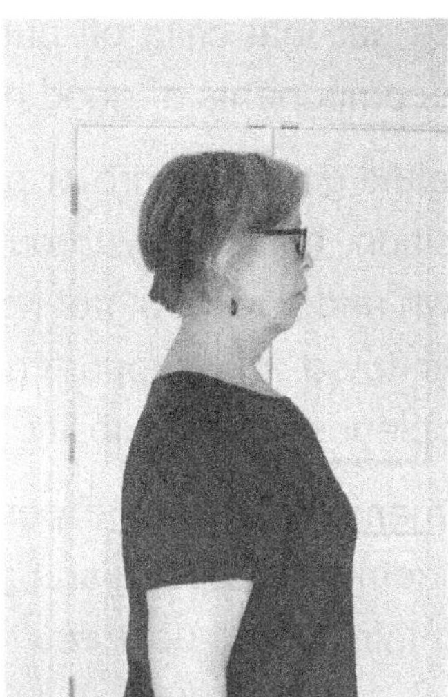

When your body is poorly aligned, as in forward head position, that bad posture negatively impacts:

- Breathing
- Digestion
- Mental clarity/concentration
- Mood
- Physical energy

Ouch!

Just reading that hurts, but it also makes me aware of my posture right now.

How about you?

Let's get that child off our shoulders and understand the components of good posture.

I define good posture or proper alignment as an open position, particularly through the chest, shoulders are down and back (but not rigidly held), head is balanced over torso and supported by the neck which retains suppleness and flexibility.

Remember that good posture is both a physical arrangement of body parts **and** a mental idea, i.e., how you think about posture.

A simple generalization for better posture is *head over shoulders, shoulders over hips, hips over feet*.

Looking from the right side of your body, optimal alignment would be a straight line from your right ear to right shoulder, to right hip, to right ankle.

Have someone take a picture of you from the side. If your body stacks properly as stated above, then yes, your body parts are aligned. If not, where do you see a misalignment?

Most of us **DO NOT** have proper body alignment, due to how much we may sit or drive, the lack of exercise and other issues. Poor posture can improve. The first step is awareness of your current posture.

Tips

Here are some tips to become more aware of your posture and to improve your posture:

- **Visual Tip** Have someone take a picture of you from the front and from the side while you're at your desk or scrolling through your phone. Is your head pulling forward and down? Are your shoulders up to your ears?

  For the side view, go through the checklist mentioned above to see if your body parts are stacking one on top of another. If not, note what body part is out of alignment. Once you know your specific habits, you can design a short routine targeted to your tendencies.
- **Physical Tip** Add easy mobility exercises for head/neck/shoulders. Shoulder rolls, shoulder shrugs, gentle neck turns, chest openers are simple to add to your day. If you're unsure what these exercises are, you can go online to check or ask a fitness professional or physical therapist. If you have physical or other medical issues, ask for advice from your doctor or physical therapist before you start any new exercises.

- **Massage** Having a supple, flexible neck is critical for good posture AND good neck movement. Neck stretches and/or massage can help. Getting a massage from a skilled massage therapist can be a wonderful way of relieving muscular tension and stress. If you have any joint or spinal issues, consult with your medical professional first.

RESOURCES

Work with a personal trainer or physical therapist to identify muscular imbalances and have them create a stretching/strengthening program to address your issues. We all have weak muscles, tight muscles, overstretched muscles. Most of us are unaware of our poor posture habits so consulting a professional can help.

Yoga teachers and Pilates teachers often include posture work in classes. Check class descriptions and teacher bios listed online. Look for a teacher who stresses proper body alignment, general mobility and flexibility.

Consider taking a private lesson with either an experienced yoga teacher or Pilates teacher to get individual attention for your body. Private lessons can be pricey, but a single lesson means the instructor's eyes are completely on you rather than scanning a class.

WORKPLACE SET UP

Evaluate your workspace.

In general, you want your computer monitor at eye level. Your hands can rest on a flat surface below the monitor. If you have wrist issues, a foam cushion which supports your wrists as you type may be helpful.

The height of your desk and of your chair matters to support good posture. Bodies vary so you may need to experiment with your set up.

Some companies offer staff the services of ergonomic experts. Accept the opportunity if your company provides this.

Ergonomic experts will evaluate your desk, chair, electronic devices and lighting as they evaluate what the right combination is for your body.

If your company does not provide this, you may find useful ergonomic information online or you can also consult a physical therapist on proper set up.

Ok, now you know what bad posture is and why it's bad for you.

Test time: Quick, demonstrate your best posture.

Did you immediately hear your parent's voice in your head yelling "STOP SLOUCHING!!!" or "SIT UP STRAIGHT!!!"

Your parents were right, as we've noted above, slouching is not good for your body.

As a child, though, you probably only heard your parents' critical comments or yelling.

Sometimes good advice is delivered in a way we can't hear, let alone act on.

Let's move past your parents and focus on you as an adult living in environments frequently unkind to your body.

Not kind:

- hours of sitting
- texting/phone scrolling
- constant Zoom meetings
- TV watching/laptop streaming
- little or no exercising
- no attention to body position (posture)
- stress

We've mentioned that bad posture can cause a host of physical, mental and emotional issues such as headaches, neckaches, shallow breathing, lack of mental clarity/poor concentration, low back and hip pain, etc.

Still not convinced you should think about your posture?

Bad posture can also make you look shorter, heavier and less energetic. Bad posture can also look defensive or weak, like when someone is startled upon hearing a loud noise or suddenly frightened.

The typical reaction is to cave the chest forward and hunch up the shoulders to protect the front of the body. If you're in an important meeting like a job interview, pitching an idea or in an evaluation with your supervisor, you want to look strong and confident. Good posture helps that. Poor posture conveys the opposite.

Worse, over time, bad posture can lead to weakened bones from poor positioning and an increased risk of falling and fractures. Your head weighs approximately 7-12lbs.

With a head forward, text-neck position, your head, all 7-12lbs of it, is now hanging off the front of your body, unsupported by the torso/core.

Take another look at this common head/chest malalignment:

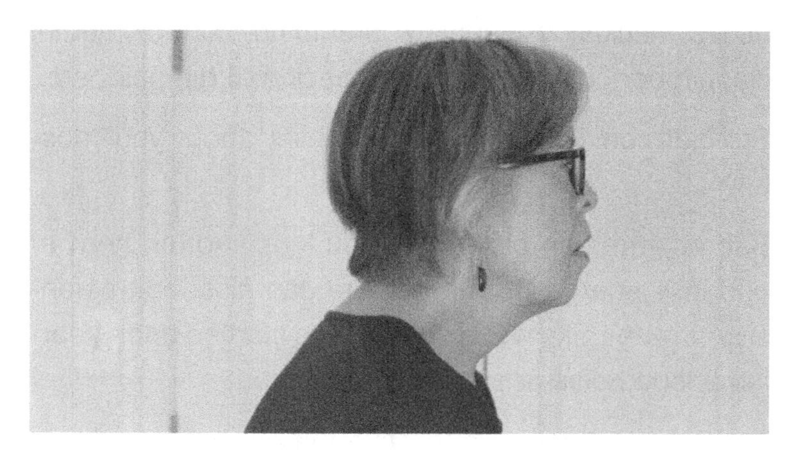

This misalignment pulls on the upper back usually causing the person to hunch forward with their shoulders and rounding the upper back to compensate.

We've previously discussed that years of a caved-in chest, rounded shoulders position could result in headaches, neckaches, upper back issues as well as potential falls and fractures.

And there's another common activity negatively influencing posture:

Looking at your cell phone while walking.

We all do it.

However, the distraction of whatever you're doing with your phone increases the possibility of a bad outcome whether that's missing a curb, tripping on an uneven sidewalk or running into someone.

If you absolutely cannot put away your cell phone, at least hold the phone higher.

Typically, we hold our cell phones at waist height or lower. To read the phone at that height, we must dip our chin down which automatically starts pulling our head forward, resulting in malalignment of our body.

If you need to check your phone, stop moving and hold the phone at eye level. Or use the audio function so you don't have to read. Then you can listen to directions or instructions and still be moving.

Next time you're out, observe people as they use a cell phone while walking.

Can you see the posture defects previously mentioned such as caved in chest, head forward and down and rounded upper back?

Those folks are one step away from a potentially serious injury.

Building Awareness

Sometimes people can sense an issue in their bodies and simply don't know how to fix it or whom to ask for help.

We can't see our head position or if we've aligned our bodies properly so there's no visual feedback as to how we're holding ourselves.

And given how much we sit and how sedentary most of us are, proper posture is not a natural state. Like breathing, until there's a problem and our bodies start to hurt, improving our posture is not high on our to-do list.

However, increasing your awareness of posture, even a few minutes a day can help change poor alignment if done consistently.

An easy way to remember to work on posture is to set an alert on your phone or laptop to take a 30 second posture break every hour or better, every 30 minutes.

Small efforts, like regular posture breaks, will pay big dividends over time.

Here are some suggestions for becoming more aware of your posture and instituting change.

Deeper Dive

MENTAL TIPS FOR IMPROVING POSTURE HABITS

- Learn what *your* posture habits are. Remember a picture is worth 1,000 words. An earlier suggestion was to get a family member or friend to take pictures of you at your computer or when you're on the phone. A front and side view will be helpful to see your specific habit.

- Based on the pictures, what do you see? Is your head or chin jutting forward? Are you slouching or rounding your shoulders? Are you caving in your chest? Identify your main issue and try some of the physical tips. Done regularly, they will help you better sense when you're slouching or reaching your head forward to look at your computer or dropping your head forward and down to look at your phone.

If slouching or any of the other less than optimal posture habits are your default position, that's what feels normal and you probably won't recognize when you do it. You need to know what better posture feels like. Feeling the difference between sitting or standing with better alignment and slouching will get clearer over time. Eventually you'll notice when you're slouching and be able to correct that posture fault.

Consistently practice new changes. As suggested previously, set posture breaks on your phone or other electronic devices. If possible, after every 30 minutes of sitting, get up to stretch or move for a few minutes.

- Recognize you will default to previous bad habits when stressed, tired or upset Remember we tend not to breathe when feeling negative emotions. If we're scared suddenly, we may exhibit a startle reflex which is a tense, defensive position with shoulders shooting up to the ears and pulling the head back.
- Change your environment to support better posture (for instance change the height of your computer, hold your phone higher to your face so your head isn't pulling forward and down to view the screen)
- Learn the difference between poor posture and well aligned posture, particularly how those 2 positions feel in your body. If you practice posture daily through the posture breaks, over time, you will be able to sense and fix poor posture more quickly. Any improvement in posture is useful.

Understand that improving your posture can be a lengthy process and requires mental and physical energy. I consistently include posture, both strengthening and stretching during sessions with my personal training clients and in yoga class.

The results are well worth your efforts.

Posture is also a component to balance. This is particularly important for older adults. I will leave it to you to define "older." This link between posture and balance will be discussed more in the next chapter.

Resource:

Review physical therapist Dr. Murat Dalkilinç's posture video:

https://www.youtube.com/watch?v=OyK0oE5rwFY

His video is a great visual for all the points made above. Plus, it's fun!

Client Story

A handbag, a backpack and a messenger bag walked into a bar

When we first met, Anna complained about neck, shoulder and lower back pain, all on her right side. Her posture demonstrated the typical "too many hours at a desk" posture-rounded shoulders, protruding head and caved-in chest.

She had seen her physician, but the doc found nothing medically wrong with her. Yet, when she saw me a few weeks later, Anna was still experiencing significant discomfort.

In addition to other fitness goals, Anna wondered if working out would improve her right-side issues. As well as addressing these right-side issues, I also wanted to address her posture.

I created an upper body program emphasizing mobility, weight training and static stretching. Anna's discomfort lessened over the next month but not as much as I had hoped.

Her right-side discomfort was a puzzle until one day when I saw her walk into the gym in street clothes. Anna's handbag was slung over her right shoulder and she was tilting sideways as she walked. When questioned about her handbag, she said she always wore it on her right shoulder and "carried only essentials."

I jokingly said her bag looked like it weighed 10lbs! Anna retorted that she thought it was 2lbs at most.

Now we had to weigh it.

Her bag came in at a hefty 8lbs.

We were both astonished.

Imagine strapping an 8lb dumbbell to your right shoulder and walking around like that for months. Picture how you might throw your handbag in the car or grab it without thinking when getting out of the car. Consider the wear and tear on your body.

No wonder Anna had significant discomfort.

Ergonomically, a heavy handbag carried constantly on the same shoulder is the **worst** choice. The weight of the handbag is not evenly distributed over the body and that shoulder never gets a break from carrying the bag.

In Anna's case, her right shoulder and right side were forced to work harder than her left side.

The heaviness of her handbag and the position of the bag (it dangled below her hip, which means it bounced a bit as she walked) caused her to elevate her right shoulder to keep the bag in place. She also listed to the right with every step. Her spinal alignment was affected as well. When she walked, her spine pulled to the right causing her body to curve/bend to her right side.

I asked Anna if she would consider alternatives such as a backpack or a cross-body/messenger-style bag. A backpack distributes weight evenly over the body and ergonomically is the best choice. A cross-body bag also distributes weight more evenly over the body and is the next best choice compared to a backpack.

Anna's answer was a resounding no.

She explained neither alternative was fashionable. Anna worked full-time and wanted what she thought was the professional look of a handbag.

Anna finally agreed to:

- Use a smaller bag.
- Shorten the strap on the new bag so it rode slightly above her hip (less bouncing).
- Get the bag's weight below 5lbs.
- Switch the bag from right shoulder to left shoulder rather than only using her right shoulder.

These changes lessened her physical discomfort and months later her discomfort was gone. With less discomfort, Anna was able to sit up and stand straighter. Over time her posture improved as well.

Ever since that day, I evaluate clients for whatever they carry on a routine basis, be it a handbag, briefcase or backpack.

I ask them to weigh their bags to assess how much they are lugging around.

Most clients are not aware of how heavy their bags may be nor are they aware of what the most optimal physical positions are to carry weight on their bodies.

Here are additional tips to prevent neck and shoulder pain caused by carrying purses and bags as reported by the American Occupational Therapy Association and the American Academy of Orthopedic Surgeons:

3 Tips for Carrying Bags

1. Always limit the weight of your bag to 10% of your body's weight. For example, if you weigh 100 pounds, you should not carry a bag that weighs more than 10 pounds.
2. At least once every month, clean out your bag. This is because sometimes you tend to carry things you don't need.
3. Because narrow straps place weight on smaller areas, choose bags that have wide, adjustable straps.

Carrying weight whether that's a handbag, groceries, a squirmy child or pet is a daily occurrence for most of us and an activity we repeat for much of our lives.

Not only do we need to consider how much that purse or laptop bag weighs but also how we are carrying it. Additionally let's consider what physical components are needed to carry weight safely and properly such as posture, arm, back and core strength.

What changes can you make to lighten your load and spare your body?

KEEP IT SIMPLE

Head over shoulders, shoulders over hips, hips over feet

Learn to feel the difference between poor posture habits and better alignment.

Correct posture as necessary throughout the day.

3 BALANCE

"A good stance and posture reflect a proper state of mind."

Morihei Ueshiba (1883-1969)
Japanese martial artist and founder of Aikido

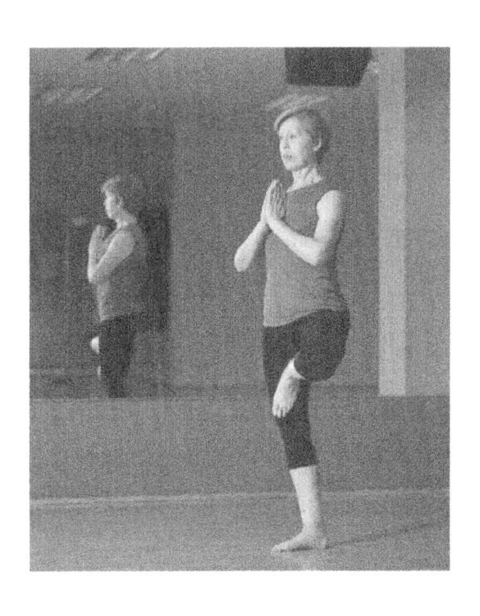

Here's a challenge:

Can you stand on one leg with the other foot off the floor, eyes open?

Be safe and if needed, put your hands on a table or back of a solid chair before trying this. It's ok to use an assist such as holding on to the chair or putting a hand on a countertop if your balance is a little shaky.

Count the seconds you can stand on one leg. Then switch legs, count the seconds and compare your times for both legs.

I'll wait.

How did you do?

Were you wobbly even with a hand down?

If you started with your hand off, did your hand reach out for the wall, a table, a chair or did you tap your foot on the floor to steady yourself?

Are you better at standing on one leg than the other?

Your answers to these questions are important information to evaluate your ability to balance on one foot.

The ability to balance whether standing or moving is critical to human life. Maintaining good balance during walking for instance, is key to staying upright and to prevent falls.

If you haven't stumbled, tripped or fallen recently, you probably haven't paid much attention to your balance. Like breathing and posture, we tend to ignore these elements of living, that is, of course, until something goes wrong.

Falling is a realistic fear, no matter your age. You already know falling can hurt.

You've probably twisted your ankle during your life or bumped into something or someone when jostled in a crowd. Maybe you escaped with a minor ankle sprain, however, serious injuries can and do occur.

Our sedentary lifestyles and the aging process put us at higher risk for injuries which could require surgery and extended rehabilitation such as a fractured hip, wrist or arm.

Head injuries may also occur from falling such as concussion or a fractured skull.

These types of injuries could affect our ability to continue living our lives the way we want, may limit our physical movement temporarily or permanently and cause ongoing pain and discomfort.

A CDC study states that, in 2020, "Among adults aged ≥65 years (older adults) in the United States, the leading cause of injury and injury deaths is unintentional falls. * Although the estimated prevalence of nonfatal and fatal falls increases with age, falls are not an inevitable part of aging. Older adult falls can be prevented by addressing modifiable risk factors through effective preventive strategies."

https://www.cdc.gov/mmwr/volumes/72/wr/mm7235a1.htm

A Johns Hopkins School of Medicine report agrees, "While it's not completely possible to prevent a fall, exercises that focus on balance and strength training can reduce the risk of falling."

According to the US Preventive Services Task Force, "The most effective programs combine activities that directly focus on balance with functional exercises (moves that resemble everyday activities, such as standing up) and strength training..."

Balance training, then, is a vital part of a movement routine for all of us.

Fortunately, by understanding the elements of balance and with daily practice and professional guidance, you can improve.

ELEMENTS OF BALANCE

While balance may seem like a fixed position, it's not. Like posture, balance is a **dynamic** alignment of your body parts when standing, seated and while moving.

If you recall from the previous chapter, posture is also a dynamic alignment of your body parts while standing, seated or moving. We will get to this link between posture and balance a little later.

Staying active, injury free and maintaining independence as we age are top goals for many seniors and reaching these goals is partly dependent on our ability to stay upright.

Let's understand the concept of balance better.

What exactly is balance?

The medical dictionary "Medicinenet" states:

"...balance is a biological system that enables us to know where our bodies are in the environment and to maintain a desired position."

According to this definition, balance has at least 2 elements:

an understanding/awareness of our body in a physical environment and the ability to maintain a desired position.

For most of us "... maintain a desired position" means standing upright in some capacity, which can include walking, running, dancing and any movement on land. Being land-based creatures, remember that our bodies are always working against gravity to stay upright.

Balance is composed of multiple body systems: your brain, vision, vestibular system, muscles, ankles and feet.

All these systems must coordinate, communicate and execute their roles properly for us to stay upright. The more complex the movement, the more vital it is for the body's systems to work together.

Please note your brain is included in this list. A key theme in this book is how to get your mind and your body to collaborate better. The idea will be explored more in Chapter 5 and 6.

If you watch a baby moving, you may notice various body parts wiggle and wobble.

The baby hasn't yet developed the strength each muscle needs to do its individual job properly. Nor is the baby's brain able to communicate and coordinate all its body parts to work together.

Maybe you're thinking, "Well, of course, a baby's mind isn't able to consciously control its body but I'm an adult and I can control my body parts just fine."

Try this little experiment and see how you do:

Standing comfortably in bare feet (or socks) with proper posture (see Chapter 2) and pick up all 10 toes.

Pretty easy, yes?

Put all 10 toes down.

Now, pick up all 10 toes and press down **just** your 2 big toes.

Put the rest of your toes down so all 10 toes are back on the floor.

Now pick up all 10 toes and press down **just** your little toes.

Put the rest of your toes down so all 10 toes are back on the floor.

How did you do? Did your toes respond?

If not, are you surprised at your inability to consciously move your toes?

We give the command to our feet and our toes don't respond. If we can move our toes at all, usually they will not move independently.

Moving your toes independently will help both your balance and walking. If you consistently practice toe raises, your toes' ability to move individually will improve.

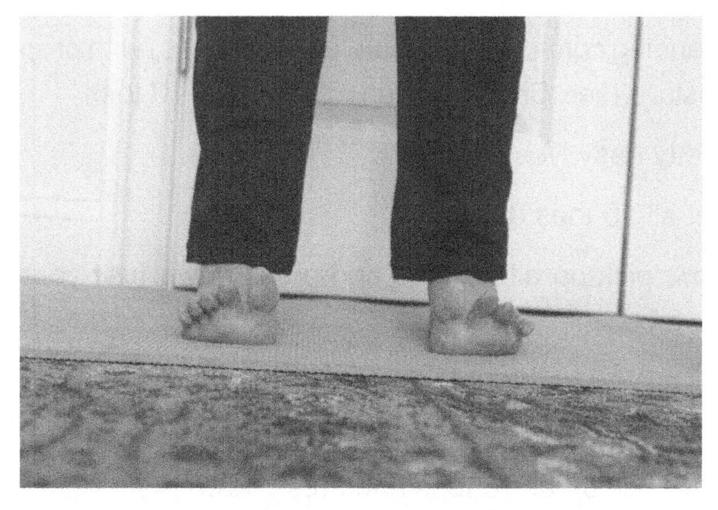

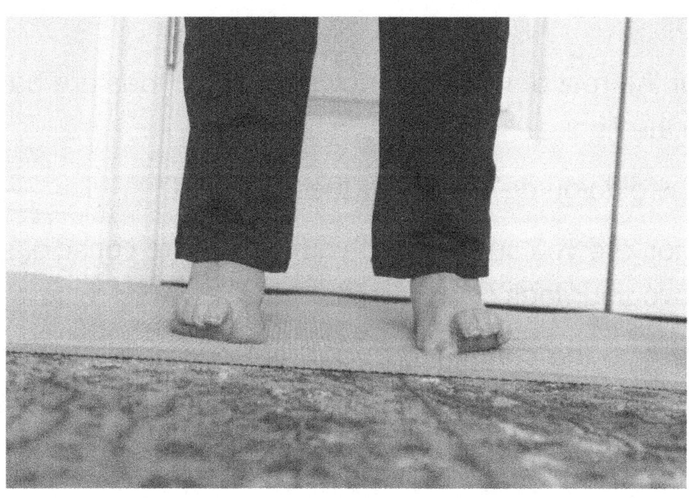

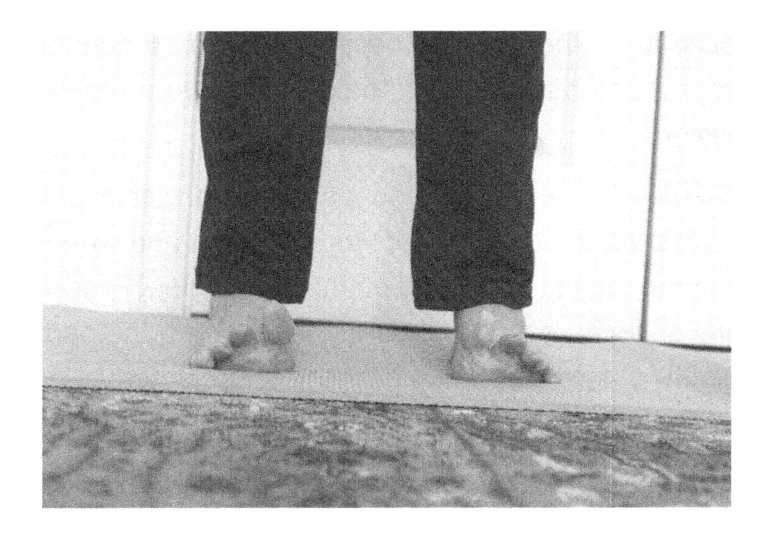

Physical Tool #1

Let's practice the single leg balance exercise again described at the beginning of this chapter. It's easy to do while you're waiting for your coffee to brew or for something to heat in your microwave. Another easy time to practice balance is while you're brushing your teeth in the morning or evening.

For safety, be near something you can put your hand on for stability. A kitchen countertop, the bathroom sink or a table will work.

Establish the amount of time you can stand with each leg off the ground. This is your baseline.

Notice if you need to start with a hand on a countertop or if you put your hand down during your practice session.

You may be able to stand on one leg significantly longer than the other leg. If yes, note that and work to lengthen the time standing on the weaker leg. Practice daily until you can stand on the weaker leg the same amount of time as standing on the stronger leg.

If you're starting with a hand on the countertop or holding onto a chair, practice taking off a finger or two for a few times and then try taking your hand off completely. Review the client story "Gail" below for more tips.

You also may find you're stronger at certain parts of the day.

Remember, safety first so make sure you practice your balance somewhere that you can grab hold of something solid if you feel wobbly.

Practice daily and keep data such as the length of time you can stand on each leg and/or whether you have a hand down or 3 fingers down. Assess yourself in a month-6 weeks and observe if your balance has improved. Can you stand longer on each leg? If yes, by how many additional seconds? Set a goal of 30-45 seconds of standing on each leg.

If you can do 30-45 seconds of single leg balance already, consult with a fitness professional or take a yoga class for more advanced balance training.

You may not be aware that your mind and emotional state also influences balance. Read on for a client story.

Client Story

Gail

A 75-year-old client hired me specifically to help her improve balance. Gail lived independently, was terrified of falling, injuring herself and being helpless on the ground.

When I asked her to stand on one foot to assess her baseline, Gail could not pick up her foot without immediately panicking (her term), tilting over and putting her hand on a countertop to right herself. She was aware that her emotional reaction (panic) and her underlying fear of falling were getting in the way of improving her balance.

Were other factors such as lack of leg strength or poor vision also at play? Yes, however, the panic she felt initially overshadowed the other factors.

Feeling panicked about falling is a reasonable response. Gail associated any attempt at balancing with panic about falling. To improve her balance, we needed to separate those two elements somehow. I was not going to logically dissuade her from feeling panicked. Instead, I focused on shifting Gail's perspective on balance to bypass her panic reaction.

I had 2 goals for Gail: 1. Increase her confidence in her ability to balance

2. Get her to understand that practicing a new skill is often uncomfortable.

I had to choose a balance exercise she could be immediately successful at to help build her confidence. In addition, I needed to help her become OK with feeling uncomfortable.

To address the first goal, I created a balance challenge that she found safe(r) than the single leg exercise described at the beginning of this chapter. Instead, I had her try a **stationary** tandem stance, sometimes called "sobriety test," meaning her right foot was directly in front of her left foot with the heel of the right foot touching all 5 toes of left foot. She used an assist as needed, for instance, putting her hand on a countertop or on a chair for more stability.

To address the second goal of getting her used to feeling uncomfortable without panicking, I asked Gail to note her discomfort, but I also asked her to notice she was still upright. Over time she realized that feeling uncomfortable did not automatically mean she would fall.

After several months' work, Gail reported less mental panic and fear of falling while doing balance exercises. Gail also discovered she could stay upright despite feeling somewhat unsteady and uncomfortable.

I gradually added more challenging balance exercises to her program, and we were able to eliminate the props.

I continue to work with Gail. Currently she can stand on each leg with better stability, without props and for longer periods of time. She is pleased with her progress and feels more confident in her abilities.

I appreciate that Gail was willing to work on a challenging physical skill colored by an intense emotional state. Our minds can be our best friends or our worst enemies.

Gail was very afraid of falling and her fear got in the way of her trying to improve her balance. She knew she couldn't change this situation by herself.

She took the step of contacting someone to help her. While Gail's fear is not completely gone, she now has tools to better manage her state of mind while still improving her balance.

Do your emotional states affect aspects of your physical ability?

The next time you're frustrated, angry or frazzled, try balancing on one leg. Or conversely try a balance challenge when you're feeling relaxed or happy.

What do you observe? Do you find it easier, harder or no difference standing on one leg in a negative frame of mind versus a positive emotional state?

I encourage you to explore how your mindset may affect your body. If your negative emotions affect your physical ability, you may be able to work with yourself like Gail did.

We'll explore this idea more in Chapter 6 "Self".

Besides your body systems and emotional states, there are other external and internal factors affecting balance.

EXTERNAL FACTORS

Let's review external factors that can pose problems for your balance:

- Gravity
- Weather
- Wind
- Ground conditions
- Slope
- Tripping hazards
- Shoes

Some of these factors are out of our control. For instance, there's not much you can do about gravity except understand that it exerts its power on us throughout our lifetimes. Because of gravity's constant force, our bodies must build stronger bones and muscles to move. When astronauts travel to space for extended periods, they experience significant muscle atrophy due to the lack of gravity in space. Astronauts exercise in space to offset this atrophy.

Gravity is not good or bad, just something to be aware of as a force on your body. Keep moving and let gravity do its thing.

Weather is a more obvious factor affecting balance than gravity. Ever try to walk or bike into a head wind or driving rain?

Ground conditions matter. Level, smooth pavement is easier and safer than uneven bricks or cobblestones.

Grass can be an issue if it is wet or isn't level. Wet grass is extremely slippery. Not good for staying upright!

Walking or running on concrete is hard on joints over time. If you're a runner/jogger, consider running on a well-maintained track rather than sidewalks which are often concrete.

Walking uphill or downhill can be difficult for those with lower body orthopedic issues such as hip or knee arthritis or weak leg muscles. Uphill ***and*** downhill can be equally challenging for different reasons.

Recommendation: if starting a walking program, look for flat, even surfaces first. An outdoor track at a local public school can be an excellent choice for outside walking. As you continue to walk and become more conditioned, you can add easy hills for more of a challenge. Be particularly mindful of walking or running downhill if the ground is rainy/icy/snowy or there's loose gravel or wet leaves.

And remember that ground conditions absolutely affect your balance when walking or running downhill.

Tripping hazards are everywhere!

Look out for:

- Curbs

- Stairs
- Uneven bricks/cobblestones/pavers
- Potholes
- Sidewalks with frost heaves
- Tree roots
- Water on the ground, melting snow, black ice
- Pebbles/rocks

These issues are largely out of anyone's control.

Let's cover two elements you **can** control.

BALANCE ELEMENTS YOU CAN CONTROL

- Inside flooring and rugs
- Shoes, sandals & slippers

At home, throw rugs, thresholds & mats can be problems. Different heights of flooring may pose a tripping hazard when walking from flat wood floors to a rug or on/over a threshold. Rug edges can often fray and corners can curl up. Consider using double sided carpet tape to tackle either issue. Or eliminate small throw rugs completely if possible.

The shoes you wear matter.

Heels, whether shoes or boots, and most backless shoes like flip flops and slides affect how your body weight gets distributed over your feet as well change how your feet contact the ground.

Wearing heels pitches your body weight forward and compromises balance by this unequal weight distribution on the front part of your foot in addition to not having the heels of your feet in solid contact with the ground.

Some clients have had their shoes slip off when walking in backless slides.

Have you ever caught the front of a sandal on the lip of a step or curb?

I have though fortunately I did not fall.

Cushy loose slippers generally do not support your feet. Those types of slippers may easily slide off your feet or worse, not provide any traction on the floor. If the floor is slick or even slightly wet, you may slip.

Clients have reported low back pain, tight calves and problems with their feet/toes after slippers, heels and backless shoes over time.

Better choices are usually shoes with a low or no heel and with backs, which can include sandals. Consult a podiatrist, physical therapist or your doctor concerning shoes and your individual situation.

INTERNAL FACTORS

As a reminder, the multiple internal factors which affect your balance include:

- Brain
- Eyes
- Vestibular system
- Core
- Legs
- Ankles/feet

Each of these must function properly AND work together as a coherent system for us to stay safely upright.

Additional factors that influence balance:

- Quantity and quality of daily sleep
- Prescribed medications
- Alcohol and/or recreational drugs
- Previous injuries or surgeries
- Medical conditions

In addition, excessive sitting and lack of daily movement may contribute to unsteadiness when attempting to stand and walk, again putting us at risk of falling.

Here are suggestions for addressing internal factors:

- Have a medical professional evaluate your balance.
- Schedule yearly eye exams.
- Use nightlights in your living space, particularly in bedrooms and bathrooms.
- Talk to your medical professional about medications you are taking that may cause dizziness or unsteadiness.
- Add daily movement such as walking or other types of exercise if safe and appropriate for you.
- Get up and move every 20-30 minutes to break up extended periods of continuous sitting. Set an alert on your laptop or phone to remind you to move.
- Practice balance daily. Standing on one leg is a good starting point and track your time. See if you can work up to 30 seconds standing on each leg.
- Implement a consistent work-out routine focused on strengthening core and legs such as traditional weight training, Pilates or other classes.
- Take yoga, Tai Chi, dance or martial arts classes. All are recognized as ways of improving

coordination, agility, balance, mind body connection and lower body strength.

- Water exercises such as swimming, pool walking and aqua classes are useful to improve balance, core and leg strength. Water is a great stress release and may increase restful sleep.

POSTURE AND BALANCE

While falling and sustaining significant injuries are common concerns, most older adults don't associate good posture with improving balance.

Let's look at examples of where poor posture negatively affects balance while moving:

1. Walking with head jutting forward. A forward head position throws off the alignment of head over shoulders. As soon as the head goes forward, the weight of the head pulls on the upper back, causing the shoulders to round forward which pulls the shoulders out of alignment with the hips.
2. Walking while looking at a cell phone (head down, "text-neck" position). If your eyes are looking down, your head will start to drop down as well. The weight of your head now pulls on your upper back, caving in your chest. Not only

are you at risk of running into someone or tripping, but you've also altered the alignment of your chest over your hips, resulting in your back working harder to maintain your position.

3. Walking with hands clasped behind the back. Even standing still like this is bad posture. To be able to hold their hands behind their backs, most people will round their shoulders forward. In this scenario, the shoulders are now out of alignment over the hips. The chest caves in and tends to pitch forward pulling the torso off the hips, disrupting alignment more.

All 3 of these flaws are posture related and negatively affect balance.

Remember the alignment generalization already mentioned, "head over shoulders, shoulders over hips and hips over feet." Alignment of body parts is crucial to staying upright.

A skilled personal trainer can design an appropriate core, leg strengthening and balance program as well as create a proper stretching/mobility/flexibility routine for you to do at home or at the gym.

Given the lack of movement and body awareness in our culture, balance training is a vital element for everyone's exercise routine.

Include posture work to improve balance.

In addition to practicing on a single leg, improving ankle, foot and toe mobility will also help your balance. Here are some suggestions for a daily balance routine.

Physical Tools

Consider these tools to be a daily balance practice which includes toe and ankle work:

Pick one or do all 4, your choice.

#1 In a standing position with good posture, knees lightly bent, pick up all 10 toes, put all 10 down, repeat 5-6x total. It's best to do this exercise with bare feet so the toes can move easily.

#2 In a standing position with good posture, knees straight, do double foot heel raises. If you have access to stairs with a railing, put your feet on the bottom step, have your hands on the railing(s) and lift both heels up, hold for a 1-second pause and lower; do 8-10 repetitions. You can do this in bare feet or wear shoes if you prefer.

#3 In a seated position with good posture, feet flat on the floor, lift all 10 toes up (leaving rest of both feet down on ground). Put all 10 toes down, repeat 4-6 times. I find this is easier done if in bare feet.

#4 In a seated position with good posture, feet flat on floor, lift all 10 toes up leaving heels on the ground, then put both feet back on the floor. Then lift both heels off the floor leaving the balls of feet/toes on the floor, put them down and repeat the entire sequence 4-6 times. Either with bare feet or wearing shoes, whichever you prefer.

Practicing standing single-leg balance is the start of the different types of balance exercises we need.

Once you've established a consistent routine of practicing your single leg balance, continue to challenge your balance in a variety of ways. The more variety the better.

We often encounter unpredictable situations as we move around in life whether that's uneven, wet ground or getting jostled on a crowded sidewalk.

Training for these kinds of unpredictable circumstances is very useful.

A fitness professional or a physical therapist can recommend appropriate balance exercises beyond the single leg balance offered here.

KEEP IT SIMPLE

Practice balance every day

Focus on proper alignment of body parts

Include posture work with balance training to maximize your efforts

4 PHYSICAL ACTIVITY

"The body will become better at whatever you do, or don't do. If you don't move, your body will make you better at not moving."

Ido Portal (born 1980) Israeli athlete and trainer

We are told incessantly that physical activity is beneficial for our bodies, our brains, our hearts, and our souls. It's true.

What may be less obvious is that continued physical activity is critical to aging well.

Some clients define aging well as not falling, being able to live independently and easily manage daily activities. Others want to feel well enough to travel and drive.

In general, most people want to feel energetic enough to live the life they choose and avoid injuries and health issues.

Take a moment and consider how you define aging well.

What's important to you? How do you want to live your life?

By now, I hope you agree that breath, posture and balance all contribute to your body functioning optimally. We know that regularly moving our bodies is equally important.

We know we should move more but sometimes even thinking about increasing our physical activity may be overwhelming.

Managing an exercise program, let alone actually working out, involves mental effort.

You may ask:

- Where can I find accurate and useful information about exercising?
- Is it better to exercise at home or at the gym?
- Should I find a group fitness app or rent a Peloton?

- How should I adapt exercises for my body and age?

Ugh.

That's too many decisions. Staying on the couch looks pretty good right now.

If you're new to exercise or haven't worked out in a while, getting started may be challenging.

If thinking about exercising overwhelms you, start with easy movements that you can do now.

Any movement that doesn't hurt is better than no movement.

Here are some suggestions:

- Walk outside around your residence if you are able and you feel safe. Aim for 10 minutes but 5 minutes will do. Depending on the layout of your residence, you can walk inside or walk up and down several flights of stairs.
- Ask friends about their exercise routines for ideas.
- Explore your community's fitness centers if available. Many towns give seniors a substantial discount on memberships and other activities. My local community fitness center costs

$60 a year with the senior discount. That's an incredible deal.

- Have a dance party in your kitchen if that's your jam.
- A morning or evening at-home yoga practice is a great way to start or end your day.
- If you're tech-savvy, there are multiple online options for every kind of movement. Many are free (YouTube), some are paid apps or subscription based.

Start. Now.

For many people, figuring out an exercise routine can be daunting. If you do an online search about exercise, you may quickly become overwhelmed with the amount and sometimes contradictory nature of information.

Instead, have you thought about how you use your body during a typical day?

Your daily activities might include:

- Walking
- Carrying books, a laptop or a purse
- Reaching for something above you
- Climbing stairs

- Pushing open a heavy door
- Getting down to the floor and back up again
- Unscrewing the cover of a jar
- Getting in & out of a car
- Turning your head to look both ways while driving
- And yes, getting up and down from your comfy couch or cushy recliner

Fortunately, practicing foundational movements directly related to these daily activities will help you get stronger and create more ease in your life.

For example, learning how to squat properly makes getting in and out of a car and up and down from a chair easier.

And no, a squat is NOT about touching your butt to the floor.

A squat is a movement done from a standing position where the squatter lowers their body **towards** the floor (not to the floor) by bending knees and hips, keeping the core engaged and chest up.

Squatting is a normal human movement, done multiple times throughout a day of normal living. Sitting in a chair and getting up again is a squat (when done properly).

Getting in and out of a car involves squatting. Using the toilet requires squatting.

If you're not sure what a proper squat is (and it does vary somewhat depending on your body), here are pictures of a squat starting from standing position to bottom position.

Remember your body is unique so your squat may not look exactly like the demonstration in these pictures.

To return to standing, push through your feet, straightening your body back up.

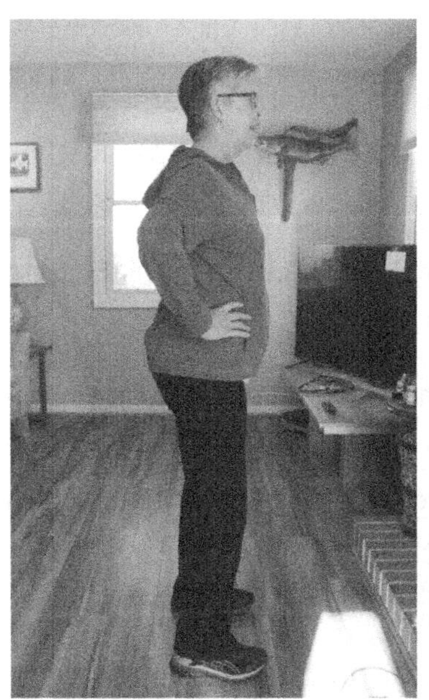

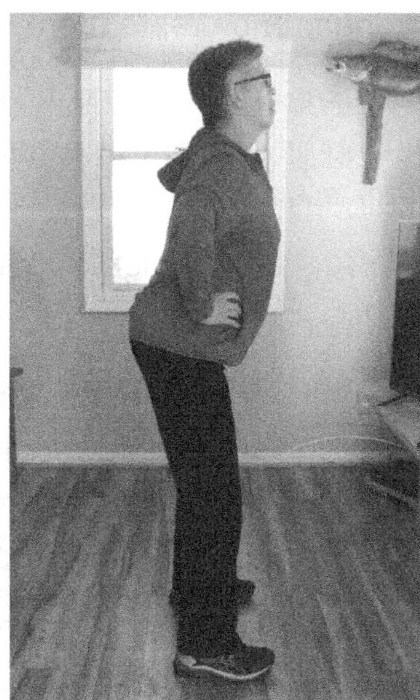

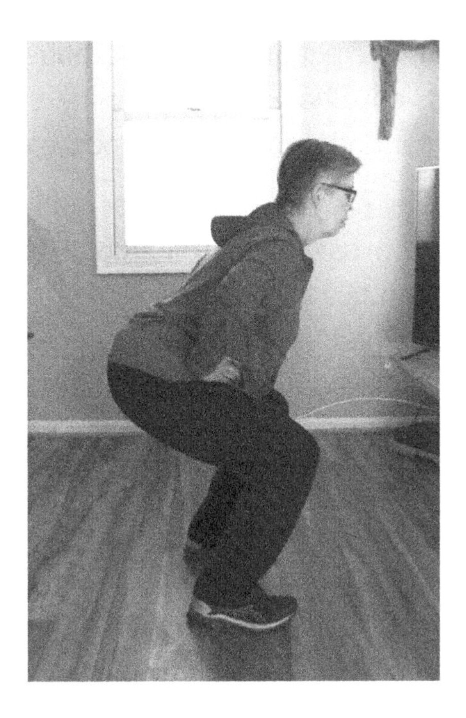

Here's a client story demonstrating foundational movements needed to do a simple life activity: Going to the grocery store.

Client Story

A Trip To The Grocery Store

Marty looked in the fridge and sighed. The milk she wanted for her morning coffee had expired. Could she skip her beloved coffee?

Sighing again, she put on her coat, grabbed her purse and went outside. She walked down the short flight of stairs to her car and drove to the grocery store.

After parking her car, Marty slung her purse across her body, grabbed a basket and searched for milk. She put the carton in her basket and remembered several other items she needed. Retrieving those extra items, Marty wished she had gotten a cart since the basket was feeling heavy on her arm. "Wait" she said. "I can do this."

Marty remembered the words of her group fitness instructor from all those classes she had taken at the local community center. She heard her teacher's voice in her head reminding her to carry weights using her core rather than her back. She also recalled the teacher's gentle but constant reminders about the importance of good posture and what good posture is.

Marty immediately pulled her shoulders down and back and lifted the top of her chest a little bit. Ah, I feel this! With better posture, I have less pressure in my lower back, she thought to herself.

She went through the self-checkout lane, bagged her groceries into 2 separate but equally weighted bags, walked back to her car and loaded the bags. She drove home and took the bags from the car. Carrying a bag in each hand, Marty carefully walked up the stairs.

She put the milk on the countertop and started brewing her coffee.

Glancing at her phone while waiting for her coffee, Marty noticed her step count was at 1,000 steps already!

"Mission accomplished" Marty said with a satisfied smile.

Marty's trip to the grocery store involved using her body in basic ways:

- Getting dressed
- Stairs
- Walking
- Squatting (in and out of her car)
- Lifting
- Carrying
- Twisting

Essential movements for grocery shopping include:

- Walk with and without weights
- Turn/twist safely

- Lift weights from a high shelf to the shopping cart or floor
- Squat properly and lift weight from the floor to a high countertop
- Go up and down stairs

Perhaps you don't give grocery shopping a second thought in terms of how you're using your body. Most of us don't until we can't use our bodies the way we want to.

Consider that some of us:

- Can't lift a bag of groceries because of a shoulder, neck or back injury
- Can't lift a heavy item off the floor
- Aren't strong enough to carry heavy bags any distance
- Are at risk for injuries due to a weak core and/or back
- Are shaky on our feet
- Worried about falling or slipping
- Can't get up and down stairs because our knees hurt and/or we get out of breath.

For some people, a simple trip to the grocery store may be a tiring and potentially unsafe activity.

It does not have to be that way!

BETTER MOVEMENT IS POSSIBLE

Practicing basic movement patterns is beneficial for most adults.

You don't need to join a gym or buy expensive equipment to do this.

You can easily find foundational body exercises online or join a group fitness class like Marty did in the above story.

Most group fitness classes include basic movements like squats.

And you don't need to work out for hours to practice the exercises.

Your program could be 5-10 minutes a day where you rotate through fundamental exercises like squats and balance one day, walking another day, core/back strengthening exercises another day, joint mobility/flexibility the next day and so on.

Think of foundational exercises as a daily health habit like brushing your teeth or washing your hands.

Boring? Maybe.

However, practicing fundamental movements regularly gets your body moving and as explained earlier, can make your daily life easier. Even practicing a few minutes daily will yield improvement. Consider them aspects of your self-care routine.

Over time, little by little becomes a lot.

CREATING A BASIC DAILY PROGRAM

There are so many ways to add foundational movements to a daily program.

Identifying your weak areas and then intelligently exercising them strengthens those muscles and can make your life easier.

Being stronger is a very good thing.

Not only does daily life become easier, being stronger may help keep you injury-free.

You may be less prone to straining your shoulder or back when lifting that carry-on luggage into the overhead bin of a plane or lifting the heavy holiday platter from the kitchen cabinet above your head onto the countertop.

Learning how to squat properly and lift a heavy item from the floor or lift something safely overhead is important!

Many of us assume we know how to do this, until that one time something goes wrong, and we end up with a serious injury.

A 5-minute core program done consistently will help you lift and carry weights safely and possibly spare your back from injury.

If you are concerned about doing exercises correctly, hire an experienced personal trainer.

An experienced trainer will discuss your goals, design a program based on them, watch you for proper form, demonstrate new exercises and guide you through your routine.

Medical clearance from your doctor may be necessary. If you hire a trainer, discuss any medical issues and physical limitations with the fitness pro including sharing what medications you take. Some medications cause dizziness or blood pressure changes and may affect your ability to exercise safely.

Your program should be individualized to you and your specific situation. Any prospective trainer needs to do a thorough medical and lifestyle intake. Trainers offer their services in gyms, online and some will even come to your home for in-person sessions.

Once you've learned some exercises and made your routine a weekly habit, a trainer will change your program with either modifications to current exercises and/or adding different exercises.

Daily life is challenging enough. Simple movements practiced intelligently (and regularly) can assist in providing more ease, peace of mind and safety in how you live your life.

And, as demonstrated in Marty's story, a trip to the grocery store gives you extra steps!

CAUTION

Many older females I've worked with are put off by the word "fitness." Though fitness, weight training and exercising are common terms, clients may view them as foreign ideas.

Additionally, these clients often feel stymied by the equipment in the gym. They don't understand how to use or adjust weight training machines. They're concerned about looking stupid and getting injured.

In fitness classes, they may encounter exercises they can't or won't do for similar reasons (hello burpees).

First, if the words "fitness," "weight-training" and "exercising" feel unrelatable to you, let's re-frame exercising to mean physical activity and fitness to mean better movement.

Let's replace "fitness" with the phrase "moving more" or "getting fit(er)."

ASK FOR HELP

Second, if you encounter a machine you don't understand, ask for help. We were all beginners once. If there's an exercise you don't like in a class, don't do it or ask for a modification from the instructor after class.

And, as a reminder, a well-balanced movement routine includes cardio/aerobic activity, weight training, flexibility/mobility/stretching, core and balance training.

Nutrition, hydration or sleep are critical elements for better health as well. However, this book only deals with the physical aspect of movement.

Evaluating what you're eating and drinking and how well/if you're sleeping are useful.

Your current physical state and ability to move well are built on:

- the nutritional choices you make every day
- the quality/quantity of daily sleep
- quality and amount of daily movement if any

If you want to have a better functioning body, consider how you're caring for it.

Some factors may be out of your control such as medical conditions, pain levels and other circumstances. Think about what you can control and start there.

And yes, you must lift weights to get stronger.

If you're not experienced with strength training, you can find online weight training programs and group fitness classes as well as apps to help you learn basic exercises.

You can also hire a personal trainer to design a weight training program individualized to you.

Remember, a trip to the grocery store involves a lot of lifting and carrying. As stated above, being strong(er) is a very good thing, particularly if you want to live independently as you age. Being strong(er) can help you in your daily life and minimize injuries if they do occur.

Whatever we call it, regular movement is vital.

AN ALARMING STATISTIC ABOUT MOVEMENT

The CDC 2020 report revealed that almost 90% of women aged 65 and older **DID NOT** meet the 2020 guidelines for aerobic and muscle strengthening activities.

Some of these women may have physical or medical conditions preventing them from daily movement.

Most do not.

That's a truly frightening figure. Some seniors are one twisted ankle away from an emergency room visit, surgery or worse.

Link: https://www.cdc.gov/nchs/products/databriefs/db443.htm

What are the CDC's guidelines?

They include:

150 minutes (2 hours and 30 minutes) to 300 minutes (5 hours) per week of moderate-intensity **aerobic physical activity**

or 75 minutes (1 hour and 15 minutes) to 150 minutes (2 hours and 30 minutes) each week of **vigorous-intensity aerobic physical activity**

or an equivalent combination of **moderate- and vigorous-intensity aerobic activity**

2 days a week or more of muscle-strengthening activities of moderate or greater intensity involving **all major**

muscle groups (usually defined as 8-12 muscle groups)

Well, ok, that's fine but if you're not exercising now, going from zero hours a week to 5 hours a week may sound overwhelming.

If you've never lifted weights, you may have no idea what your major muscle groups are, let alone know how to exercise them.

It does sound intimidating and confusing.

Let's break down the CDC guidelines into something more manageable.

Here are some suggestions.

Mental Tip #1 Start where you're at

Assess your current physical state. If you're not moving regularly, what type of movement is possible for you?

As has been said in this book, walking, even 5-10 minutes daily, is a great start to improve your aerobic activity as well as your mental health. Peer-reviewed research shows "a positive, statistically significant relationship between exercise/physical activity and mental health."

Reference: Mental Well-being in the Fitness Industry Inspire 360 Global Fitness Newsletter Issue #15, May 2024 IDEAFIT

If weather or safety are issues, consider walking inside. I have clients who walk the halls of their high-rise apartment complexes and others who walk in enclosed malls to get their steps. Maybe you prefer biking or swimming or a group fitness class. Go with whatever you find interesting. Any (safe) movement is better than no movement.

MENTAL TIP #2 Build Consistency

Is 5-10 minutes enough?

Sure, to start.

If you haven't been moving regularly, it's better to consistently be moving every day rather than moving a lot one day and not moving at all for the next several days.

Build a daily habit. Once you view your 5-10 minute daily walk as a regular part of your day, add more time, perhaps another few minutes. If walking feels like a chore, think about listening to music, a podcast or audio book as you walk.

Will walking with a friend will make your walk more enjoyable?

RESOURCES

If you haven't done weight training for a while or not at all, as mentioned previously, take an in-person or online beginning group fitness class or hire a trainer to teach you.

You don't have to join a gym unless you want to. During the pandemic, many personal trainers began offering online services. Some also created apps, which for a small monthly fee give you access to fitness routines. The same is true for dance, yoga and Pilates.

There are online resources ranging from useful to ridiculous to downright harmful. Read the comments and reviews before you try the work-out. Consult with your health care professional before starting a new exercise routine.

If you haven't worked out or moved regularly in months or years, start slowly, learn proper form from a professional and as mentioned about squatting above, don't expect your body to look exactly like the instructor's or class members' bodies.

You may not know what is right for you until you try; however, taking a 90-minute advanced class when you haven't worked out in months is inadvisable at best.

If you want to join a gym, that is certainly an option. Every health club has a "vibe" so evaluate whether you would be comfortable working out at the club.

Most gyms offer a complimentary single day or week-long pass. Take advantage of that, if offered, to see if you like the gym's atmosphere.

The vibe can change depending on whether the club is quiet or busy, so ask the staff about peak hours if that matters to you.

Again, consult with your healthcare provider for their professional recommendations. Certain exercises or kinds of exercising may not be right for you depending on your personal situation. Medical advice is **always** a good idea before starting a workout routine.

When you start/restart a consistent movement program, you may be surprised with the 'musical' accompaniment your body makes during exercising.

Your joints are often the featured soloist in this scenario. Here's Jamie's experience.

Client Story

A Symphony of Sounds

Jamie began her squat exercise and a symphony of sounds ensued.

"Click!" went her left knee. "Snap!" sang her right ankle. "Crackle!" bellowed her left hip and "Pop!" trilled her right shoulder.

How many sounds can human joints make?

Apparently, many.

Joint noise during exercise may seem alarming but these sounds are often attributed to air or other gases popping when the joint moves.

Dr. Timothy Gibson, MD, orthopedic surgeon and Medical Director of the Memorial Care Joint

Replacement Center at Orange Coast Medical Center in California says, "A painless crack or pop is normal, as long as it doesn't hurt or produce swelling, it's nothing to worry about."

A quick online search shows that Dr. Gibson's comments seem to be the prevailing medical opinion.

Jamie agrees. Her clicks, snaps, crackles and pops don't bother her and she's never noticed any joint swelling. Rather than disturbed by the abundance of sounds, Jamie's appreciative that her joints still move without pain.

Jamie isn't my sole client whose joints express themselves.

Some other clients also hear loud joint noises during exercise.

Knees are a favorite place for popping, but any joint can sound off. Ankles may crack during yoga class, hips pop while stretching, elbows may click doing an overhead press. Some folks may feel “crispy crunchies” in their necks during yoga class or while doing neck mobility exercises and stretches.

There’s even a fancy term (or a depressing one, depending on your outlook) for joint noises - “crepitus.” It comes from the Latin word for “a rattling, crackling noise, a creak.”

The English word “decrepit” is derived from crepitus and, according to *Oxford Languages*, decrepit means “elderly and infirm.”

However, the Cedars-Sinai website has a similar view to Dr. Gibson, stating, “clicks, pops, snaps, crackles “do not necessarily signify advanced age” (whew!).

The site adds that “the sounds MAY be a sign of arthritis, cartilage wear or an injured joint.” So, if your joints produce multiple noises during exercise, assess for pain and swelling. If in doubt, consult your medical professional.

And like Jamie, perhaps be grateful that your joints are still able to move without pain even if during exercise, your body "composes" a symphony of sounds.

https://lnkd.in/gQufMrSk

https://lnkd.in/gkGCTaC8

As We Age

"A body in motion stays in motion;
a body at rest stays at rest."

Isaac Newton (1643-1727) English Polymath

A client recently asked if he should be walking 10,000 steps a day for the rest of his life.

Great question.

Our bodies change as the years pass but the need for movement does not.

Movement, strength, power, breath, posture, flexibility and mobility are all important physical elements to maintain, to live life the way you want.

My answer, then, is yes and no.

If walking 10,000 steps is possible, it's safe physically and walking gives you pleasure, then absolutely continue walking.

If you're the type of person who, if you don't reach 10,000 steps, views that as failing to meet your goal, then change your expectations.

For instance, if walking 10,000 steps seems impossible, consider rephrasing the goal to walk every day, maybe for time rather than actual number of steps (10 minutes? 30 minutes? More?).

Do something and be consistent.

Celebrate whatever movement you accomplish, rather than dismiss your efforts.

CAUTION

The goal of walking 10,000 steps **is not** a magic number.

In fact, it was a marketing tool devised to promote a Japanese made pedometer ahead of the 1964 Tokyo Olympic Games.

Surprised? I was.

If you're interested to learn more, read this informative journal article for a fascinating look at how the idea of 10,000 steps was created: Tudor-Locke, Catrine & Hatano, Yoshiro & Pangrazi, Robert & Kang, Minsoo. (2008). Revisiting "How Many Steps Are Enough?".

Medicine and science in sports and exercise. 40. S537-43. 10.1249/MSS.0b013e31817c7133.

While continued research makes the benefits of more steps rather than fewer steps very clear, your step count is also dependent on other factors you can't easily control such as weather, safe walking routes, schedule and time constraints, etc.

As you may have already surmised, a major theme of this book about movement is starting where you're at and then be consistent with what you're doing.

If your daily step count is fewer than 10,000 steps, consider ways to increase your walking, like adding another 500 steps.

As mentioned above, a trip to the grocery store can easily amount to 1,000 steps, depending on the size of the grocery store and how much you walk around the store.

There are health benefits to more steps rather than fewer steps but if you don't reach 10,000 steps every day, you have not failed!

Any movement, including walking, is better than no movement.

Earlier recommendations are to start small, repeat often and consistently. Once you have a habit of moving, you can consider other options for different kinds of movement.

Start with success: what can you do now?

Remember Gail's story in Chapter 3?

Gail's balance was significantly impaired, and she was concerned about falling. We started with what she could do - balance on one foot with a hand on a countertop.

Then she went to several fingers on the countertop instead of her entire hand and worked, slowly over time, to standing on one foot without any assistance.

Establish what you **can** do. Then, build on that.

And we'll take a deeper look at failure in Chapter 6.

CONSISTENT MOVEMENT

While more overall steps may result in greater health benefits, remember that consistent daily walking is an excellent place to start moving, regardless of your step count.

I suggest walking because humans are designed to walk. But any movement is useful like dancing, swimming or using a cardio machine such as an elliptical in a gym.

Whatever you decide, your exercise program needs to be specific to you and address any medical or physical limitations.

I've had clients who continued exercising through all stages of life and with many kinds of health and physical issues.

The oldest client I've had to date was 103 and was legally blind. She participated in daily exercise classes including strength training and balance until the end of her life.

Again, do what's possible for you now. Look to maintain your present level of fitness and then aim for a little bit more whether that's another 5 minutes of walking or another day of weight training or adding a yoga class or whatever your more might be.

You may be inclined to dismiss the idea that a small increase is not good enough but over time that little extra movement you do every day adds up.

Your extra movement or added weight training or yoga class may mean the difference in how you live your life by avoiding falls and preventing injuries.

RECOVERY

Besides breathing, posture, balance and physical activity, recovery is another key component to keeping your body healthy.

Were you aware that when you lift weights, you are breaking down the muscle tissues you're using to lift the weights?

While that might sound like a bad idea, be assured it's the first step to strengthening your muscles.

The second step is recovery. And this is an element many of us overlook.

Recovery means giving muscle tissues a chance to rebuild themselves to be stronger and more resilient.

You may have heard that you shouldn't weight train the same group of muscles 2 days in a row.

This is why.

Here's a simplified example: If you're doing bicep curls for instance, by lifting weights, you're breaking down your bicep muscles.

Your arms require at least 48 hours to recover i.e., rebuild the tissue which was stressed by the bicep curls. If you don't allow for proper recovery and choose to do bicep curls again the next day, you are essentially breaking down already broken-down tissue.

Not a good idea.

Recovery means time between strength training as in the example above, but rest, sleep, easy movement (light yoga, walking or stretching for instance), foam rolling, massage or other types of body work are also part of recovery.

As we age, recovery becomes even more important as it takes an aging body longer to recover from exercising than a younger body.

USE IT OR LOSE IT

You may have heard the term "use it or lose it" in reference to exercising, meaning if you're not moving, you may lose the ability to move. To a degree, this is true.

If we don't maintain a regular movement routine, the aging process means we lose significant muscle mass resulting in less strength and power.

Less strength and power affect balance, to name one physical element, so we are less stable on our feet, increasing the risk of falling and possibly getting injured.

The aging process also affects our metabolism which slows down, making any weight loss goal more challenging. Additionally, hormones change or cease causing other health issues.

We can't control many of these bodily processes. However, regular movement may help minimize some of the effects of aging.

The bottom line is that, to function well, our bodies need movement throughout our lifetimes.

But strike a balance between intelligent exercise and necessary recovery. Both are critical to keeping your body moving well.

KEEP IT SIMPLE

Move. Frequently. Now.

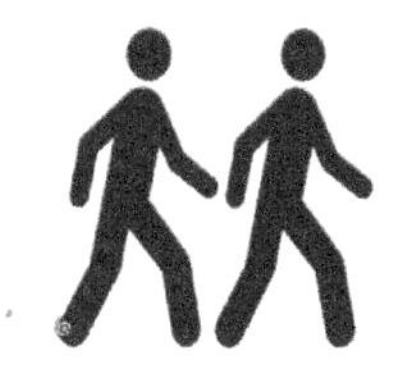

5 MIND

"be softer with you.
you are a breathing thing.
a memory to someone.
a home to a life."

— Nayyirah Waheed, Poet & author "Salt" (2013)

How does your mind contribute to the puzzle of moving your body more and better?

Every day you make many small decisions concerning, among other things, moving, feeding and resting your body.

These decisions, made consistently over time, help create the body you will have in a year, two or five.

You are literally making your future body now.

I often say to clients,

"You are either your best friend or your worst enemy. You get to decide.

What's your decision?"

Ask yourself:

Does your mind function as a capable partner with your body? Or is it an oblivious bulldozer, pushing the body past its limits, not providing enough rest, healthy food or water?

In the daily rush of life, many of my clients focus more on checking off items on their overflowing to-do list than on listening to their bodies.

A single day of not listening might be manageable, but eventually the body will rebel against being mistreated and ignored.

Are you listening when your body tells you it needs more movement, better sleep or more nutritious food?

You've probably heard or read the phrase "mind-body connection."

We frequently encounter this idea in wellness articles, yoga and Pilates classes.

It's a wonderful concept about staying present to your body, whether that's focusing on your breath or on the physical sensations of your body as you're moving.

My interpretation of the mind-body connection expands the common definition to include how well your mind and body work together in service of whatever goal(s) you want.

In this book, that's movement and self-care.

I'm advocating taking a wider view to include the many decisions you make daily concerning your body.

How well do you use your mind to help your body move forward, literally and metaphorically?

Your mind can sabotage your best efforts or collaborate with your body.

If you pay attention to how you direct your body and the decisions you make that affect your body, you can begin to better understand, listen for and interpret the body's signals.

A closer, more productive relationship means you can make intentional choices about movement and self-care rather than reacting without thought or simply pushing through life.

KEEP IT SIMPLE

How do you live in your body?

THE JOURNEY

"To plant a garden is to believe in tomorrow."

Audrey Hepburn (1929-1993)

Dutch-British Oscar-winning actress, fashion icon

If you wish to incorporate more movement in your life, then you're in a change process and desire some sort of result or goal, in this example, more movement.

You have a gap between where you are and what you want.

The process of bridging that gap is the journey.

Audrey Hepburn's quote above, "To plant a garden is to believe in tomorrow." is similar to setting a goal and then acting on your intentions.

When you plant a garden (set a goal), you believe that the garden will eventually bear fruit i.e., change and results are possible.

Why else plant a garden?

To create a garden, you must have a clear intention and take action.

But planting a garden also means that there is no guarantee the garden will produce the fruits of your labor.

While you may believe or hope or have faith the garden will yield results, ultimately, you do not control when or if the garden blooms.

Belief, hope and faith are not enough to get results from either a garden or your goals.

Let's raise the odds.

Here are suggestions about how to establish a goal and then how to better endure the journey and reach your destination.

1. WHERE ARE YOU?

"Wherever you are is the entry point."

Kabir (1440-1518) Indian mystic poet & saint

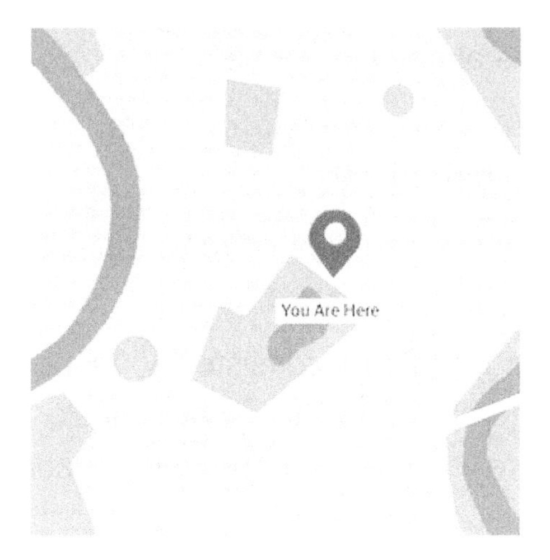

Vecteezy.com

Kabir's quote, "Wherever you are is the entry point" recommends you start where you are. If you know the starting point, then getting to where you want to go is much easier.

A useful analogy may be the maps that indicate "You are here," usually accompanied by a red pin or other symbol.

The pin orients you.

You must know where you are first and then you can establish where you want to go.

Clarifying your starting point can save you getting turned around or headed in the wrong direction when you embark on the journey of reaching your goal. If you want to go north but you are unknowingly facing south, you're already in trouble.

Let's use the map example of "Here" to mean your current daily movement.

If you're getting minimal or no movement, *that's* where you are now. It's your "Here."

If you go to the gym inconsistently, *that's* your starting point. If you spend hours at a desk, sitting with poor posture and having frequent headaches and backaches, then *that's* your baseline. If you've fallen in the last year, *that's* part of your entry point.

Tip

Describe as accurately as possible your average day in terms of movement, breathing, posture or balance. Write it down or think it through in your head. This is your "Here."

CAUTION

Your starting point will differ from that of others. Please, no comparing and no beating yourself up for realizing you're in a place you don't want to be. No self-blaming or self-shaming allowed.

Remember Waheed's quote:

"you are … a home to a life."

Treat yourself nicely, as if you're welcoming a cherished guest into your home.

KEEP IT SIMPLE

Plant a garden (*aka* believe in tomorrow).

Know where "Here" is.

Be gentle with yourself.

2. DATA

Business management expert **Peter Drucker** said, *"You can't manage what you don't measure."*

I agree.

Applying this concept to movement means knowing the numbers that represent your starting point, your "Here."

For instance, if your goal is to increase daily movement, then it's useful to know your *current* walking average or daily step count. It's your "Here."

Tip

We live in a digital age, which provides abundant information. For example, most smartphones, smartwatches and smart rings can track your steps. Specialized fitness trackers can give you the same information.

You increase movement by taking more steps than your current daily average. And yes, taking 5 more steps **is** more. *You* get to decide what more is.

Track your progress over time.

No, you do not need a spreadsheet. As we said, if you wear a smartphone, smartwatch or smart ring when you walk and the device is on, the numbers automatically register.

Your smartphone or fitness wearable is your virtual assistant AND your accountability coach.

If you know how many steps you took the previous day, it becomes much easier to equal or exceed that total today.

To track your exercise data, use a virtual calendar or an old-school, hard copy calendar to record if you exercised. Next, observe your progress over time.

To track your weight training routine, such as noting type of exercises, total weight lifted, sets and repetitions, buy a weight training log or simply use a notebook.

You could keep a weight training journal with your smartphone as well.

Bottom line: collect the data.

PROGRESS

Noting your progress is an extra step.

But tracking data allows you to see progress which is very useful on the journey towards your goal.

In the daily busyness of life, we rarely stop to notice our progress. But tracking progress is **critical** to generating momentum. As you will read below, momentum is a close companion to motivation.

After a walk or an exercise session, look at the progress you've made on your smartwatch. It can be very helpful (and motivating) to review your data at regular intervals.

And celebrate **all** your progress, no matter how small. Be your best cheerleader and give yourself a big pat on the back for whatever progress you make.

And if you don't see progress, reviewing your data can give you a much clearer picture of what's not working and provide clues as to why.

For example, perhaps you overestimated how many times you walked the previous week. By reviewing your data, you can see you missed 2 of your 5 sessions.

Missing 2 sessions isn't that big a deal for one week but over time those missed sessions add up.

If you don't track your data and review your data regularly, you won't know.

KEEP IT SIMPLE

Track data to establish your baseline.

Review the data regularly.

Celebrate all progress. Often. Yay, you!

3. WHERE DO YOU WANT TO GO?

Would you set out on a trip without knowing your destination?

To some of you that might sound like a fun adventure.

That's ok if you like meandering, potentially going in circles or possibly not arriving anywhere.

If that scenario doesn't appeal to you, then it's vital to know where you want to go.

Otherwise, you may find yourself in the same situation as described in *Alice in Wonderland* when Alice asked the Cheshire Cat for advice:

Alice: Would you tell me, please, which way I ought to go from here?

The Cheshire Cat: That depends a good deal on where you want to get to.

Alice: I don't much care where.

The Cheshire Cat: Then it doesn't much matter which way you go.

Alice: ...So long as I get somewhere.

The Cheshire Cat: Oh, you're sure to do that, if only you walk long enough. Is that what you want?

To get somewhere? Anywhere?

Then any map will do. Even if it's the wrong map.

Save your valuable energy.

Don't be Alice.

You need a map.

The first step is knowing where you are.

The second step is knowing where you want to go, aka, setting a goal.

SETTING A GOAL

What's your goal?

There are many types of goals, such as short-term and long-term goals, and many methods for setting goals.

Work with goals whatever way is best for you.

A good rule of thumb is to write them down.

Again this may seem like an extra step.

And, like collecting data on walking or other exercise, it is.

Still, these steps are vital.

Once you've clearly identified your goal, you are in a much stronger position to know how to set appropriate action steps to achieve your goal.

We'll get to action steps shortly.

First, here is a suggestion on setting goals:

Set a short-term goal that you think you can accomplish easily.

Several advantages of short-term goals are:

- you can progress in a relatively quick amount of time.
- they usually are more doable.
- success can generate momentum (continued action toward a current goal and/or willingness to set a different goal).
- completing a short-term goal may encourage you to tackle a bigger, more challenging long-term goal.

Deeper Dive

When setting a goal, consider one that excites and scares you a little. A goal that's a challenge and somewhat out of reach.

Goals test your abilities, physically and mentally, and promote growth overall.

Are you thinking: *Who wants to engage in a process that tests my abilities? Isn't life hard enough without more challenges, struggles and tests??? Who cares about growth?*

I understand.

Most of us prefer what's familiar, safe and predictable. We want a stable, unchanging life.

Fine.

But consider the following:

First, life is changing endlessly, whether we want it to or not.

Second, staying with the familiar and safe will not get you what you want since what you want is something you currently don't have.

Thomas Jefferson (1743-1826), third US president and author of the "Declaration of Independence", said,

"If you want something you never had, you have to do something you've never done."

Goals, by their nature, mean change. And change requires effort, growth, discomfort, struggle and doing something, probably, many things, you've never done.

Remember you have a gap you're trying to bridge. That gap is full of unknowns.

I hear you yelling: *Where's that damn remote? Time to park myself on the couch and binge on the latest reality show.*

It's ok.

You have the choice about whether to set a goal or not, of course.

But you're a lot more capable than you think and *you can do hard things*.

Yes, to be sure, the process of learning a skill or trying a new thing is often uncomfortable, particularly for adults who think they already know whatever they need to know in life.

That's a limiting belief but it allows people to stay in their comfort zone.

However, being uncomfortable is usually worth the effort as you discover that, in fact, you can accomplish something you couldn't do before.

Being uncomfortable and eventually succeeding strengthens your self-confidence and self-efficacy, the belief that if you did it once, you can do it again, whatever "it" is.

Success not only sharpens your skills but also changes how you look at yourself, your self-identity. We'll discuss that idea more in Chapter 6, "Self."

TIMING

But before setting a challenging goal, consider this:

If your plate is overflowing, the time may not be right to set a huge goal or possibly *any goal.*

How much brain energy do you have? How much time will you need in your schedule to accomplish this goal?

How much effort and money will it cost?

For instance, if you want to join a running club that meets 3x a week for an hour but you're working crazy overtime on a big project, is it wise to join that running club now?

How will you create space in your schedule to handle the hours you're working AND tack on an additional 3 hours per week for another activity?

Would you be ok with one run a week with the club? Or instead, how about running with a friend?

You have options. But considering other choices takes valuable brain energy.

When we're stressed, we often don't see beyond extremes: either we go to the running club 3x a week or not at all.

When we're at our max capacity, we often retreat to survival mode, put our heads down, grit our teeth and say, "I'll join the running club **and** work 60 hours a week," rather than acknowledging now is not a good time to add one more thing.

Consider what being kind to yourself might look like in this scenario instead of forcing your way through life.

Another thought about timing: some people will say that timing is never right.

Life is often so full, overwhelmingly full and overflowing, that the thought of adding something pushes us over the edge. In that situation, the time will never be right for whatever change you want.

I agree in principle.

If you find yourself in this state of mind, consider what you can say no to, what you can eliminate in your life to create some extra energy and space.

We'll talk more about saying no in the next section.

In addition to evaluating where you might be able to find valuable time and energy, I suggest you let go of needing your goal to happen exactly the way you envision it.

PERFECT IS THE ENEMY OF DONE

Can you think of your journey to your goal as a **general destination** rather than a highly detailed guidebook?

For example, when you plan a trip to the beach, do you pick in advance the spot you want to set up your beach chair? Do you expect the umbrella you rent to be your favorite shade of blue?

Does the weather have to be hot but not too hot?

In other words, do you need your goal to happen exactly as you want it to?

In general, it's useful to consider details when setting a goal.

However, insisting on controlling the specifics of your journey and how your goal might happen tend to lead to disappointment and the possibility of not reaching your goal at all.

There are multiple factors involved in reaching a goal. Some you can plan for but many you cannot anticipate or even conceive of.

Life has a way of throwing curve balls at us, particularly when we think we have the perfect plan.

Sometimes good enough IS good enough.

Progress is not always a continuous straight line up.

Progress, like the stock market, is often a rollercoaster, going up and down and sometimes even veering sideways.

If your actions get you even a bit closer to your goal, *over time*, you are progressing.

For example, are you moving? Good, keep going.

Done is better than perfect.

KEEP IT SIMPLE

What's your goal?

Be ok with uncomfortable

How's the timing?

Perfect is an illusion

Chasing after perfect will keep you stuck

4. ACTION STEPS

Let's assume you know where your "Here" is and you have an idea where you want to go.

How do you bridge this gap to get from A to B?

Action is key.

For instance, if you're not moving now, beginning to move regardless of the amount, is an appropriate action step. If you're moving inconsistently, then more consistency is a good action step.

An appropriate action step to increase consistency might be to move in a more scheduled fashion (a walk, an exercise class or online yoga, for instance) 3x a week.

Maybe identify the days you'll walk or exercise, say Monday, Wednesday, Friday.

Or, an appropriate action step is to identify the time of day you'll exercise, such as first thing in the morning or right after dinner.

The point is *you* get to decide.

Based on where you are and where you want to go, ask, "*What small action step can I do immediately?*"

Pick one.

The easiest, simplest action step is usually the best choice.

Do it (now, if possible), then repeat that step consistently over time.

Remember the equation in the introduction to this book?

Knowledge + Consistent Action/Over Time = Results

In "Mind Your Movement," we've reviewed basic information on human movement-breath, posture, balance and physical activity. This book includes a wide array of action steps you can take to be more active in your daily life as well as mental tips.

You have enough knowledge. To get results, **now** is the time to act and then **continue acting**.

Pick one simple action step and repeat that over time.

Progress happens with repeated action.

Track your progress.

Seeing progress tends to encourage additional effort, which produces more success, eventually generating self-belief and self-confidence.

More self-confidence gives you the mental strength to continue with your current action step or try a different, perhaps bigger, action step.

Doing one action step over time will result in progress. You define what progress is, but, please, have realistic expectations.

CAUTION

MANAGE YOUR EXPECTATIONS

If you haven't exercised in years, expecting to run a 5K next month is probably unrealistic. If you want to improve your balance, inconsistently working on balance will probably not result in observable progress.

You wouldn't be human without expectations, but please, focus more on moving forward by taking one small(er) action step, done successfully.

Manage your expectations so that the process of reaching for your goal is one small success followed by another small step, followed by another success which starts to generate momentum.

MOMENTUM

Momentum is one of your best friends on the road to any goal and it helps support motivation.

Isaac Newton's first law of motion states, *"A body in motion stays in motion, a body at rest stays at rest."*

Yes, it takes effort to add more movement to your life.

However, once you **start** moving, if you **keep** moving, it becomes **easier** to **continue** moving.

That's the definition of momentum: *"strength or force gained by motion or by a series of events."* (Merriam-Webster Dictionary)

You may need to exert considerable effort, thought, and energy to get yourself moving toward your goal, but if you keep going, you will exert less effort over time.

Each time you practice your single action step, it becomes easier. Over time, that action step may even become a habit.

For instance, walking regularly starts to require less thought and effort and eventually becomes part of your daily routine, like brushing your teeth or making coffee.

Once you start seeing results from a specific action step, as stated above, most of us are more motivated to continue.

Relying on staying motivated becomes difficult over time.

But adding small action steps that result in ongoing success becomes a winning and more importantly, a sustainable formula.

Here's a generalization about momentum:

Action + Success = Momentum = more action + success = more momentum, etc.

Success is vital to creating momentum. When you act and that action yields a positive result (however you define positive), you will be more likely to continue, creating more and more success.

This process, repeated over time, improves your self-belief that you are capable of change.

You have more agency in your life, more self-confidence and belief that you can set a goal and have success.

If you have a large goal, break the goal down into smaller, more manageable parts so you can succeed immediately with one tiny piece of the goal. Repeat this process of creating and reaching small "sub-goals" until you achieve your overall large goal.

In the beginning, working in this way may feel very slow but at some point, you will notice progress.

And momentum will kick in and you'll pick up steam.

A big goal is just many, many small goals strung together.

Little by little becomes a lot over time.

And success can invigorate you, keep you motivated and committed to achieving more.

Noting success is important. Acknowledging your progress produces momentum because you can see that your efforts are making a difference.

If you're tracking your data, you can measure how much progress you've made.

If you review your data and see improvements, you know that **you are the driving force behind your progress**. This is powerful information.

Knowing you have agency, i.e., the ability to change, increases your self-confidence.

To paraphrase Newton, once you start moving, it's easier to continue moving **IF** you *keep* moving.

That's the beauty of momentum. It's compound interest for your life.

Take one tiny action you can successfully accomplish now.

Repeat.

KEEP IT SIMPLE

Pick one simple, easy action step in support of your goal.

Start now. Repeat. Repeat again.

Practice + Repeated Action = Progress

6 SELF

"How You Do Anything Is How You Do Everything"

Cheri Huber (c. 1944-)
American meditation teacher and author

There's a long-standing adage that the only constants in life are death and taxes.

Everything else is change, change and more change.

I'd like to add another constant: you.

You bring yourself to every situation, every person you encounter, every job you work, every place you live. And you bring yourself, your personality traits, to how you move and to your self-care.

So, how's your self-awareness?

You've probably heard the idea that if you continue to have the same problems in life, even though the people in your life change, the common denominator to those problems is you.

Do you know the acronym "PICNIC"?

It means: Problem In Chair, Not In Computer.

The point is **any goal you want to achieve involves you.**

Who, exactly, then, are you bringing to the party?

Cheri Huber's workbook, "How You Do Anything Is How You Do Everything," states that each person has a degree of consistency in their actions and behavior.

What about you?

What consistent traits do you exhibit?

If you know yourself well, the answer may be obvious.

You have a great sense of humor and/or are an optimist. Perhaps you're book smart and/or have common sense. You're quiet, you're extroverted. Or you're artistic, athletic, a math whiz, etc.

We can go on and on.

Take a moment to think about your strongest character traits. You may want to make a list.

If you're not sure, here are 2 ideas:

1. Look back on your history. Notice when you felt successful or achieved a goal. How did you succeed in that situation?
2. Ask trusted friends or family what they've noticed about your strongest character traits. Before asking, though, make sure you can hear their comments.

CAUTION

ABOUT FEEDBACK

What kind of feedback do you want? What information would be most helpful to you?

If you don't make clear what you're looking for and ask for what you want, you may get feedback that isn't helpful, leaving you feeling confused or worse, criticized.

"I don't like it."

"How can you do THAT?"

"You can't do that."

"WHAT ARE YOU THINKING?"

These might be possible replies if you don't specify what type of feedback you're looking for from family and friends.

Family members oftentimes have very strong opinions and their feedback may feel judgmental.

In requesting feedback, would you prefer comments specific to what you need, phrased in a way that's supportive and gives you space for your ideas and thoughts or unfiltered, uncensored advice about whatever you're considering?

Some of us prefer warmer, more subtle comments, others want the unvarnished truth (truth at least according to the person giving feedback).

The point is, figure out what is best *for you* and then ask for that type of feedback.

You want feedback that helps you and doesn't leave you feeling criticized, diminished or stupid.

Remember Waheed's poem from the beginning of Chapter 5, be soft with yourself.

Choose carefully whom you ask for feedback.

THE USE OF SELF AWARENESS IN SUPPORT OF YOUR BODY

Did you gather your list of personality traits?

Great!

Now, how do you use your self-awareness in service of your body?

Here are some examples:

If you're someone who doesn't like crowds, going to the most popular group fitness class may not be a pleasant experience.

Maybe the thought of a 90-minute yoga class is unimaginable for you but a 20-minute stretch routine seems ok.

Think about what aligns with who you are and what type of environment makes you feel most comfortable.

If you're an introvert, you may want to start exercising at home or go to the gym during less busy times.

Certainly, after you start moving regularly and feel more confident, you may decide to try that large group-exercise class.

If you're a morning person, exercising immediately after getting up is a good option for you.

Figure out what you need and see if that works for you. You can always try a different tactic if needed.

ACCOUNTABILITY

Let's say you know where you are, you're tracking data, you've set your goal but you're struggling with consistency, what do you do now?

Create some kind of accountability system.

For instance, if you need support or accountability, ask a friend to walk with you, take a yoga class together or meet you at the gym.

Working with a fitness professional like a personal trainer offers built-in accountability by having regularly scheduled training sessions.

A favorite group fitness class can also provide accountability since it's generally held on the same day and time.

What kind of accountability do you need?

For some clues, ask yourself what's worked in the past to help establish a new behavior?

Knowing your consistent traits and being self-aware helps your mind and body cooperate.

"who are you? (Who are you? Who, who, who, who?)

I really wanna know"

The Who, from the song "Who Are You?" 1978

Have you asked yourself lately: Who am I?

You want to capitalize on your personal traits.

The first step is knowing what they are.

1. Change

"There is nothing permanent except change."

Heraclitus (c 540 BCE - c 480) Greek philosopher

"Success is stumbling from failure to failure with no loss of enthusiasm."

Winston Churchill (1874-1965)
British Prime Minister and author

Change means doing, feeling, being, thinking something different than before, which alters you in some respect or possibly many.

Working toward a goal is the same idea. While it's possible your goal may be something you've done before, when most people set goals, it's something they haven't accomplished previously.

In any case, a goal by its nature involves change.

If you're still not convinced, let me ask, "Has your goal ever worked out exactly as you thought it would?"

Are you laughing?

I think you'll agree that rarely, if ever, happens.

Goals can be defined as things we desire in life. We want to attend a certain college or be offered a particular job. We want to pass the bar or win an athletic event.

We want to lose weight, improve our movement and better manage our stress. Learn another language, travel abroad and buy a home.

Goals can be small or extra-large or any size in between.

We achieve goals through a series of actions that lead (hopefully) to the desired outcome. We can then say we reached our goal.

Sounds simple, doesn't it?

On paper, maybe, but the process of reaching your goal requires learning and, to paraphrase Thomas Jefferson's quote, acquiring new skills and abilities.

New means change.

Taking steps to reach your desired outcome alters you, sometimes in major, life-changing ways.

Change is a trickster. You may feel great enthusiasm toward your goal, fired up to succeed no matter what. This is behavior often displayed in January each year.

Then your child gets sick or your mother falls and breaks her hip or your boss assigns you a huge, 3-month project. Or you're getting married soon or divorced or returning to school.

Any number of life events can potentially derail you.

Or your goals require new skills.

Learning new skills involves practicing where, I guarantee, you will make mistakes. For every 2 steps forward; you may take 4 steps backward.

Learning something new is a process, an often frustrating one.

But you are not failing as you learn.

Learning is a natural part of setting goals and acting on them.

We'll talk more about failing better shortly.

Here are some other thoughts to consider as you move toward your goals:

UNINTENDED CONSEQUENCES

Robert Merton (1910-2003), the American sociologist, stated "actions of people ... always have effects that are unanticipated or unintended."

Merton popularized the idea of unintended consequences which I paraphrase as not being able to predict how *you* will change, even if your goal is clearly defined.

Here's an example:

Let's say your goal is attending a group fitness class 2x a week.

Perhaps attending that class cuts into time spent with your work crew at happy hour. You get pushback from your work colleagues and then you debate giving up the class. Or you keep attending the class but your happy hour friends stop inviting you and you start to feel a decided chill at work.

Or maybe you meet people in the class who become friends. They invite you on walks or to join other classes. Now your social group has expanded, but you spend less time with family and other friends.

Or you like the class so much you fantasize about learning to teach it until one day you talk to the teacher.

Or taking the class makes you realize you're getting stronger and maybe training to run a 5K isn't such a crazy idea after all.

I see these possibilities as "unintended consequences" and they're part of reaching a goal.

You can't predict what unintended consequences will occur or how big or small they will be.

But you can be certain, from your original action, other things will happen.

Unintended consequences tend to sneak up on us.

While they're neither positive nor negative, the surprise of an unintended consequence is often a bit unsettling. It's how we handle their presence in our lives that matters.

But friction can occur when unintended consequences affect our self-identity, changing our previous behavior.

SELF-IDENTITY

If you were someone who enjoyed relaxing on the couch after work, but now you walk with friends instead, you are creating a new routine which also starts to affect your self-identity.

You're no longer a "stay at home, relax on the couch after work person," but instead becoming a "walker."

If you repeat your action step for a long period, i.e., walk with friends consistently, it becomes part of who you are.

Changing your self-identity can lead to additional unintended consequences as stated above. Your identity as a walker may mean you consider doing a charity walk or taking a trip that includes a lot more walking and hiking than what you've done before.

Being a walker may result in you feeling stronger. You may start walking faster and farther. Now your self-identity includes being a "strong walker."

Viewing yourself as a "strong walker" may mean you reconsider how much alcohol you consume during happy hour since you don't like how you feel the morning after and that affects your walking.

Somehow your new self-identity as a "strong walker" becomes more important than your previous self-identity "attending happy hour with co-workers."

Continuing to pursue your goal (more movement) may produce a cascade effect of unintended consequences, a shift in your self-identity and a change in your normal patterns of behavior.

Can you have both self-identities? Is it possible that you are a "strong walker" and "attends happy hour"?

Yes.

Though at some point, those 2 self-identities may collide and you'll need to make a choice.

Which identity will you prioritize?

CAUTION

Changing your self-identity not only influences how you view yourself but how others view you, particularly family and close friends.

Some may not be keen about your changes and you will get resistance from people who don't want you to change.

Hopefully, you'll get a lot of support and encouragement from the important people in your life as you make changes to move more and better.

But be aware of mixed messages.

If you share your intention to exercise, your family and friends may initially be supportive. Eventually, though, some people may give you a hard time when you leave for your new exercise class or for a walk.

When people realize that your new goals are changing your typical behavior or social patterns, they may wonder if this new behavior will change your relationship with them.

This may be why family and friends verbally support you but sometimes seem to undercut your desire to change. They may encourage you to skip class so you'll stay with them instead and watch the latest online movie.

Your sister might say mom misses you, so you should call her now instead of taking your evening walk.

People are often fearful of what change means to their relationships.

Strangely enough, sometimes the person giving the mixed messages is us.

We may be aware that other peoples' reactions are not wholly positive, and this realization could prevent us from being consistent with our intent to keep moving.

If a friend or loved one protests because you now spend more time away from them, you may have trouble embracing your new self-identity.

Not only can your relationships with others change, as stated before, but your relationship with yourself may change also. It can be scary and disconcerting to view yourself differently.

Here's a story about self-identity and changing your self-perspective.

It's also a story about not letting other people label you.

CLIENT STORY

DENISE

Athlete: a person who is trained or skilled in exercises, sports, or games requiring physical strength, agility, or stamina.

Merriam-Webster Dictionary

When I told Denise, a 62-year-old female, that she had a lot of athletic ability, she laughed uproariously. I, on the other hand, was serious.

She dismissed my comment and with it, any possibility of viewing herself as athletic. I was fascinated and a little disheartened by her response.

In the few months since we started training, I noticed when I demonstrated and explained how to do an exercise, Denise was able to coordinate her body to perform the movement properly the first time. She was very physically strong from the beginning and was able to tackle more complex moves much sooner than other women I trained.

I had previously asked her if she participated in organized sports growing up or danced. Her answer was no. After college, she married a career military man and raised 3 children while frequently moving cities as well as countries due to her husband's postings.

This lifestyle left little time or opportunity for Denise to exercise.

After her children were grown and out of the house, she started exercising and sought out personal training to manage stress, lose weight and better control/ improve her medical issues.

She had no idea that she had physical capabilities, nor did she embrace them after I pointed them out to her.

Over the years, I've had a few other clients like Denise who never participated in organized sports but who also had physical talents such as body awareness, coordination, power, strength, stamina or agility.

When I shared that their abilities were "athletic," they were equally amused and dismissed my comments immediately.

It broke my heart a little that they were so quick to limit themselves.

Clearly being called athletic seemed ridiculous to them. They wouldn't even consider the idea.

What makes an athlete?

I'm guessing that most of us would say an athlete is someone who trains and participates in organized sports and athletic competitions.

Some of us might only include elite-level athletes as part of their definition, such as Olympic gymnasts, track and field stars or figure skaters, for instance.

They spend hours in the gym or ice rink, on the track or in the pool working to get better and better at their sport.

Is the only kind of athlete someone who trains hours a day and is super fit?

In other words, to many ordinary folks, athletes may appear unrelatable, although we often enjoy watching them compete.

The Merriam-Webster Dictionary states that an athlete is:

"...: a person who is trained or skilled in exercises, sports, or games requiring physical strength, agility, or stamina."

Well, that's interesting. There's no mention of training for hours a day, 5% body fat or washboard abs.

Are all of us who move our bodies regularly athletes?

Denise was just beginning to exercise, so while she was not yet "trained," she certainly was skilled. Her athletic skills were not utilized in her earlier years, but they were there, to some degree, in her body.

And while she hadn't participated in organized sports, as a mature woman she was exercising and starting to discover what physical abilities she possessed.

Is this important?

Her dismissal of my comment about being athletic meant she, at that moment, did not include this quality or trait in her self-identity.

In other words, since she viewed the idea "athlete" and "athletic ability" as far outside her realm of self-identity, she went to the other extreme and didn't view herself as having any physical ability.

In fact, her view of herself was "non-athletic," out of shape, overweight and medically unhealthy.

Had Denise been able to entertain the idea of having some physical ability she might have been excited to discover this new part of herself.

Maybe she would have felt more empowered in her body and more motivated to see what she was capable of physically.

Sometimes family members label children as "the smart one," "the pretty one," "the popular one," the "science geek" etc. As adults we may have a difficult time exploring different identities if we get stuck with a label from childhood.

Even if Denise only tried on this different self-identity, it might have broadened her world, opening her to new possibilities.

Fortunately, her story has a happy ending. Despite her "non-athletic" label, Denise did well with her training and was able to lose weight, get fit(er) and better control her medical issues.

Rather than athletic, her self-identity shifted to "regular exerciser," which worked for her.

And in the end, that's all that matters.

As for me, I could see that when I called Denise "athletic," I labeled her. The label didn't fit how she viewed herself and so it wasn't helpful.

As a result of that experience with Denise, I began to rephrase my comments about clients' athletic abilities and simply shared with them: "You're strong here, you're fast in that exercise, you're well-coordinated, flexible, etc. ..." rather than labeling them.

I learned to gear feedback to what my clients could hear and accept. If I had done that with Denise, she might have gotten to a point where "athlete" was a self-identity she could entertain. Or not.

What about you?

What labels do you use to describe yourself? Are they accurate?

Are you open to connecting to a new part of you?

Working toward any goal means change.

And change includes unintended consequences, which often shift how you look at yourself.

Yes and No

Setting a goal means saying yes (obviously to the goal) ***AND*** saying no.

You will face situations that get in the way, and you will need to say no to move forward to your goal.

Remember the happy hour example?

That's one scenario where someone with a new self-identity has to say no either to herself or to others.

If you attend happy hour and indulge, you may decide to sleep in and miss your next day's yoga class. Yet, if you skip happy hour, then your friends may be upset when you cancel.

Many of us don't like saying no.

Is this you?

We want it all. Happy hour *and* yoga! Yoga during happy hour!

It's an unpleasant fact that we can't have it all.

Here's where learning to be more comfortable saying no becomes important.

If you don't have a positive connection with saying no, then one idea is to change your perspective a little.

Can you view no as a useful word? It's short and to the point.

You don't have to justify or qualify your no. Of course, you can if you want, but very few people are owed an explanation for *your* decisions.

If you are uncomfortable saying no, the first couple of times that word comes out of your mouth, you'll probably encounter resistance (friends and family are notorious for testing).

But stand firm.

If you prefer, practice with less important decisions first or with strangers or acquaintances rather than close family members.

Tip

A SUBTLE NO

Evaluate those to whom you have the most trouble saying no. Perhaps you can say no in a less direct fashion than a straight out "No!"

Here's an example of a very soft no:

When I was an employee in companies and given extra assignments, I would ask my supervisor for guidance on which items were the highest priority and the timeframe in which she wanted the work completed.

Which items needed to be finished first and by when?

Given that information, I would know which assignments I could set aside and which needed attention now.

This tactic, while not a direct no, was a way for me to better manage my workload and maintain an effective working relationship with my supervisor. These were very important professional goals for me at the time.

Having my supervisor agree to the order of assignments and timelines also helped me feel less overwhelmed when given additional work.

Can you think of other ways to say no without using the actual word?

DEALING WITH OVERWHELM

Prioritizing and establishing timelines are still helpful strategies in my life.

When life is too full and I'm overwhelmed, I assess what's most critical to accomplish today.

If I'm feeling really stuck, I'll pick one small action step to do now, maybe something that could take me 5 minutes to accomplish. Remember the previous tip, "start with success?"

Having a tiny action step I can do in 5 minutes gives me a sense of success, that I've done something.

Oftentimes that little success motivates me to do more (this is the beginning of momentum). Now I feel somewhat less overwhelmed and that I've done something productive.

Change IS hard. It takes effort, time and brain energy. To say yes to your goal automatically means you must say no in other parts of your life.

Learning to say no, in whatever way you choose to, is necessary on your journey toward your goal(s) as well as incredibly useful in life.

So, before setting goals and heading out on the road, be aware of unintended consequences, self-identity pivots and the need to say no.

Otherwise, you may encounter unhappy surprises.

2. FAILURE

"Ever tried. Ever failed. No matter. Try Again. Fail again. Fail better."

Samuel Beckett, (1906-1989)
Irish writer, from "Worstward Ho" 1983

I want you to fail better.

What? Why would anyone want to fail BETTER?

Before you run screaming for the hills, consider that the journey toward a desired goal automatically means you will experience success AND failure.

If you learn to tolerate failure as well as enjoy success, you will be in a much stronger position to achieve other goals throughout your lifetime.

You will be more resilient and better able to overcome challenges and obstacles. You will also build your self-confidence and create a solid foundation to attempt new goals.

Learning how to fail better means focusing more on the process rather than on the outcome or results.

Learning to fail better could result in staying more emotionally centered and suffering less if you can have the perspective that failure is not a personality defect.

Instead, see it as information.

Can you view failure as a signpost that reads "WRONG WAY"?

Here's another analogy: failure is compost where the many scraps of learning experiences provide important nutrients for future growth.

Redefine failure the way you want that allows you to learn from the information rather than be flattened by the experience.

Normalize failure as something to be expected in a learning process like reaching for a goal.

And if you do get flattened (it happens to all of us), remember this Japanese proverb:

"Fall down 7, get up 8."

KEEP IT SIMPLE

Failure is information-redirect your efforts.

Failure is an event, not a personality trait or a fatal flaw.

Get up one more time than you fall down.

2. Success

"The road to success is always under construction."

Lily Tomlin (born 1939) American actress, comedian, writer, singer and producer

While failure is not often viewed kindly, success may also present challenges.

Think about it.

What happens when you achieve a goal? Most people would term that a success.

However, upon arriving at their destination, sometimes people experience a letdown.

Sometimes they can't believe their journey is complete. They may ask, "Is this all there is?"

These are normal reactions.

You may feel a range of emotions at the end of your journey.

When you've expended time, energy, money and effort to reach your goal and that journey is complete, you may wonder what to do next.

Even after achieving your goal, you may not feel completely satisfied with the outcome.

Maybe you didn't reach your goal exactly the way you wanted. Perhaps achieving your goal took longer than you expected.

Or you had an idea of how you'd feel at the end but that didn't happen.

It's ok to acknowledge your feelings and still recognize your accomplishment.

Remember unintended consequences?

In addition to feeling happy after achieving your goal, an unintended consequence may be feeling negative emotions as well. That mixed bag can be confusing and unsettling.

We might expect fireworks and roses at the end of our process. Life tends to be more complicated than that.

Can you be ok with feeling a range of emotions?

Here's a suggestion if you experience conflicting feelings after attaining a goal.

Tip

Notice all your feelings upon reaching your goal. Reflect on how you've grown, changed, and believed in yourself to keep going. Give yourself time to digest the completion of your journey and acknowledge any less-positive feelings in addition to the positive ones.

If you feel a let-down or other negative feelings, dig in and explore why you might feel this way.

Sometimes disappointment or frustration point to areas that still need kindness and support.

Here's another piece of my story as an example:

The first time I lost a significant amount of weight, I thought my life overall would also change. Of course, I felt better and my health improved substantially but some of the relationship and body image issues I had prior to my weight loss remained.

My life didn't automatically become sunshine and rainbows after I accomplished my weight loss goal. And those issues became much more glaring since my major goal (losing weight) was done. That was a shock and a disappointment. I sought help during this time.

Consider talking to a mental health professional to help you explore and understand your feelings in a safe environment.

What's Next

If, instead, you've accomplished your goal and you feel great, what happens now?

For me, I celebrate the conclusion of my journey first. I take time to reflect on where I started, the challenges and obstacles I overcame, the people who helped me and how I've changed.

I journal regularly so one way I reflect is rereading my journals. I also have friends and family who are willing to share with me what they observed as I worked toward my goal. Their comments give me another perspective about my journey.

At some point, I consider new goals.

And off I go on my next adventure.

SUPERCHARGE YOUR JOURNEY

"Success is not final; failure is not fatal:
it is the courage to continue that counts."

Winston Churchill (1874-1965)
British Prime Minister and author

Before you create a goal and get on the road, consider these last two ideas to supercharge your journey.

COURAGE

"Feel The Fear and Do It Anyway"

Book (1987) Susan Jeffers (1938-2012)

American psychologist and author

Surely, we can recognize, even if we're feeling reasonably positive, how much energy it takes for us to get moving and continue moving. When we feel discouraged, unsupported or disheartened, moving may feel impossible.

We can see how negative feelings may literally weigh us down, crush momentum and halt progress.

However, when feeling defeated, are we aware how courage can uplift and sustain us on the road to our goal?

Courage doesn't mean lack of fear or a heroic act.

As Susan Jeffers states above, "feel the fear and do it anyway."

When all you want is to stay in bed with the covers over your head, having courage means *doing* something, even if that something is throwing off the covers and getting out of bed.

You literally must put one foot in front of the other to get yourself moving.

Working towards a goal, not knowing what the outcome will be, how our self-identity may shift or how we'll deal with challenges and obstacles are acts of courage.

Give yourself more credit.

Setting a goal and venturing out on this unknown journey of change **is a courageous act.**

I applaud you.

It's easy to get stuck and feel overwhelmed when faced with an unexpected obstacle or challenge. You may not have the experience or skills to deal with whatever is in your way.

You have a choice to act or not, to be courageous or stay stuck.

What small step can you take now to deal with the situation?

You don't have to have all the answers. That first step you take might be wrong. And that's ok.

Mistakes are information, remember?

If your step was in the wrong direction, try again in a different direction.

This book is about information, tips and tools to help **you**.

Your courage is yours. Your goals are yours. Your journey is yours.

Do it your way.

Be Kinder To Yourself

"I've decided to be happy
I've decided to be glad
I've decided to be grateful
For all I ever had

...

I've decided to be open
To that little voice inside
Telling me I'm beautiful
It's ok to be alive"

From the song, "Kinder" (released 2004),
Copper Wimmin American Women vocal group

Many of us, me included, grew up during a time focused heavily on "self-improvement." Enormous numbers of self-help books detailed the seemingly infinite ways we needed to be better, do better and look better.

While some of the advice in these books may have been helpful, the continuous focus on what's wrong with us also contributed to self-criticism, shame and sometimes self-loathing.

Shaming and belittling ourselves to change **does not work** for most of us.

Shame and blame do not motivate me.

Does it work for you?

From letting a number on the scale or a dress size define me in years past, I am now appreciative of what my body can do, how strong I can be, how far I can walk and how I move.

Now, I am also kinder to myself. Meaning, I appreciate what my body does for me today and how hard it tries to do what my mind asks it to do. I monitor my self-talk and censor negative words and thoughts.

When I'm not happy with how my body is moving, rather than criticize and berate myself, I consider what I want to be different and take steps to change.

Mostly, all the body parts work well. And I am truly grateful for that.

"Sometimes carrying on, just carrying on is the superhuman achievement."

Albert Camus (1913-1960)
French philosopher and author

KEEP IT SIMPLE

Goals = change

Change can be uncomfortable, messy and exhausting. Keep going.

Expect unintended consequences and self-identity adjustments.

Strengthen your ability to say no.

Failing is information, not a character flaw.

Celebrate successes.

Acknowledge all your feelings.

Supercharge your journey with courage and kindness.

7 CONCLUSION

CHOICES

Autobiography in 5 Short Chapters by Portia Nelson

I

I walk down the street. There is a deep hole in the side-walk I fall in. I am lost … I am helpless. It isn't my fault.

It takes me forever to find a way out.

II

I walk down the same street. There is a deep hole in the sidewalk. I pretend I don't see it. I fall in again. I can't believe I am in the same place but, it isn't my fault.

It still takes a long time to get out.

III

I walk down the same street. There is a deep hole in the sidewalk. I see it is there. I still fall in ... it's a habit. My eyes are open I know where I am. It is my fault.

I get out immediately.

IV

I walk down the same street. There is a deep hole in the sidewalk.

I walk around it.

V

I walk down another street.

From the book "*There's a Hole in My Sidewalk: The Romance of Self-Discovery*" (1977) Portia Nelson (1920-2001) American popular singer, songwriter, actress, and author.

Can you relate to Portia Nelson's words?

I certainly can.

If you want change in your life, whether that's moving better or positive self-care, challenges and obstacles occur. Portia Nelson calls them, "potholes."

As expressed in this book, change means new. And new means you can't predict where a pothole will appear if you'll fall into the pothole or how you'll get yourself out when you do.

Well, that sounds grim.

Read Nelson's words again.

Do you see how you have choices in dealing with inevitable potholes?

If you fall in a pothole, will you stay in the pothole? That's a choice.

Can you learn to recognize an upcoming pothole and avoid falling in? It's a choice to learn.

Will you take a different street? That's a choice.

For most of us, continuing to move is a choice.

And the choices you make now, tomorrow, next week, next month lay the foundation for the body you will have next year and into the future.

But, for now, you have today.

Investing in yourself by moving consistently and regularly will eventually pay dividends over time.

Take yourself seriously.

You count. You matter.

You're worth it.

So tell me, what's your choice?

Movement Is Life So Let's Get Moving~

I'd love to know your thoughts.

If you'd like to share, email me through the contact page on my website Stiff To Fit: https://stifftofit.com

Acknowledgements

Thank you to my personal training clients and yoga class members past and present. Working with you on your movement and fitness while accompanying you through the ups and downs of your lives has been and is an honor and privilege. Without you as clients, there's no me as a fitness professional. You provided the raw material upon which the book is based. I hope you recognize the threads of our training sessions.

Thanks to my family: Greg and Margaret, David and Kathy, Martha, Carole, Elizabeth and Linnea, Spencer and Barbara. We are a small but mighty group! I'm happy we're family and even happier we're friends.

I honor these family members who profoundly influenced me and who have passed- my parents Doris & Leslie Dow, extended family Vivian & Wilfred, Ina, Art & Cora as well as honor my late dear friend, Nancey and my late ex-husband, Gary.

Thanks to my teachers, colleagues and friends in the fitness, yoga and Pilates world. I was very fortunate to begin my fitness career in Northern California, a hub of high-level health clubs, cutting edge fitness concepts and amazingly talented fitness professionals.

Moving to the metro DC area furthered my career with additional opportunities in fitness and leadership. I added kettlebells, yoga, Pilates and wellness/nutrition coaching to my toolbox and accepted leadership positions as Fitness Director at several metro DC health clubs.

My time as Fitness Manager and Director of Residence Life at several retirement communities in Northern Virginia and Western Massachusetts also deepened my understanding of healthy aging, wellness and how important movement is for every age and level. I learned an enormous amount from my experiences and am grateful to everyone who crossed my path.

My earlier musical career contributed substantially to my life overall and provided me with many skills which I transferred to fitness.

Vital skills from music included learning the value of consistent action over time (also known as practicing). Practicing taught me that continued intelligent efforts could yield positive results, an idea I emphasize as a fitness professional with my clients. Little by little becomes a lot over time.

Another vital skill learned from music is the idea of precision, playing the right note at the right time with the right sense of flow, phrasing and musicality. The need for musical precision directly translates to instructing my clients on proper form to stay safe and how to get the most out of their exercising.

While I never played an organized sport, as a musician, I did learn the importance of teamwork. Playing in bands, orchestras and in chamber music groups throughout my childhood and adult life taught me to know when to blend and when to stand out, when to follow and when to lead, what my role was at any given moment during a rehearsal or performance and how to support my colleagues and conductor well. This skill translates to how I work with my fitness and yoga clients. My clients and I are a team, and we work together collaboratively. It's also how I wrote this book, as a conversational, collaborative venture between author and reader.

Thanks to my former flute students, music colleagues and flute teachers. Being a musician in Boston was incredible. I studied and worked in a rich environment with world class music schools, performing organizations, composers and flute makers. I treasure the personal and professional relationships I made in music.

Thanks to the Alexandria Economic Development, Arlington Economic Development, Revby Small Business Consulting, Freshy Website Designs and the Latino Economic Development Center teams. As a female owner of a small business, I've been the beneficiary of grants from these organizations for website development and branding, promotion and marketing plans for my writing. Each business coach I worked with provided encouragement, wise insights and useful recommendations.

Thank you to Jessica Wolf and Dr. Murat Dalkilinç for your fantastic breathing and posture videos and for your gracious replies to my emails asking permission to use your work in this book.

Thanks to my photographers, Tori Fuller and Matt Mendelssohn. Tori, I appreciate the action shots and videos you took for demonstrations of different movements in the book. Matt, thanks for a great author picture, our photo shoot was a dream.

Thanks to my graphic designer, David Deakin for creating my book cover, spine and back cover. Your insightful comments about this book demanded I develop a more artistic eye. I now have a greater understanding of fonts, book bindings and color. I'm grateful for such amazing "in-house talent."

Thanks to my long-time business coach, Jody Kennett. I am so appreciative to have found a business coach who also understands the ins and outs of the fitness world. Having this common ground from the beginning of our coaching together has been and continues to be invaluable.

Through our monthly Zoom calls and annual in-person visits, Jody's gentle and perceptive comments helped me clarify my goals and determine appropriate steps on how to achieve them. Our yearly lunches exploring Vancouver's abundance of delicious Japanese restaurants has been such a treat.

Thanks to my editor, Seth Arenstein. Seth is a consummate professional, skilled in all aspects of writing and editing. As someone both knowledgeable about and with personal experience in classical music, exercise and yoga (to name just a few of his multiple interests), Seth offered insightful comments, pointed questions and oftentimes a different perspective, all of which I greatly valued.

Working with Seth on this book felt like a meaningful conversation with a friend who gave wise advice and whose feedback was always on point. He has made this book overwhelmingly better, though he is not responsible for any errors which are clearly mine.

Lastly thanks to everyone who read one of my articles, blog posts or versions of this book. Your comments, encouragement and support mean the world to me.

Made in the USA
Monee, IL
06 October 2024

67282975R00115